The Mother's Manual of Children's Diseases

by

Charles West, M.D.

ADVERTISEMENT.

I have often asked myself whether it would not be possible to give in a small compass, and avoiding all technical detail, such an account of the diseases of infancy and childhood, as might be of use and comfort to the intelligent mother.

Returning now, with health perfectly restored, to practise my profession for the rest of my life exclusively in my own country, I have brought with me this little book, in which the comparative leisure of my enforced sojourn at Nice has enabled me to realise my purpose.

The book is not intended as a handbook for the nursery; many such exist, and many of them are of great merit. Neither has it the worse than idle pretence of telling people how to treat their children's illnesses, without the help of a doctor. Its object is to give a description of the diseases of early life, such as may help a mother to understand something of their nature and symptoms, to save her from needless anxiety as to their issue, and to enable her wisely to second the doctor in his endeavours for their cure.

CHARLES WEST.

55 HARLEY STREET, CAVENDISH SQUARE. August 1, 1885.

CONTENTS.

breathing -- Rules for examination as to these points -- Signs of absence of disease of the brain

CHAPTER III.

General management of disease -- Mothers who cannot nurse their children when ill -- Importance of truth and keeping child happy -- Rules for management of bed-room and bed -- The bath -- Poultices -- Leeches -- Cold applications -- Medicines -- Note-taking and relation to the doctor

PART II.

PLAN PROPOSED TO BE FOLLOWED

CHAPTER IV.

On the disorders and diseases of children during the first month after birth -- Still-birth -- Premature birth -- Imperfect expansion of lungs -- Jaundice -- Ophthalmia -- Scalp-swellings -- Ruptured navel

CHAPTER V.

Disorders and diseases of children after the first month, and until teething is finished -- Infantile atrophy -- Rules for artificial feeding -- Management of indigestion -- Thrush -- Teething -- Affections of the skin -- Eczema

PART III.

DISORDERS AND DISEASES INCIDENT TO ALL PERIODS OF CHILDHOOD

GENERAL CHARACTERISTICS OF SECOND PERIOD OF CHILDHOOD

CHAPTER VI.

Disorders and diseases of the brain and nervous system -- Their mortality and its causes -- Convulsions -- Congestion of the brain -- Sunstroke -- Water on the brain -- Inflammation from disease of the ear -- Chronic water on brain -- Brain disorder from exhaustion -- Spasmodic croup -- Epilepsy -- St. Vitus's

THE MOTHER'S MANUAL

OF

CHILDREN'S DISEASES.

PART I.

INTRODUCTORY.

CHAPTER I.

ON THE MORTALITY OF CHILDREN, AND ITS CAUSES.

The purpose of this little book will probably be best attained, and needless repetition best avoided, if we begin by inquiring very briefly why so many children die, what general signs indicate that they are ill, and what general rules can be laid down for their management in sickness.

The first of these inquiries would be as useless as it would be sad, if the rate of infant mortality were fixed by determinate laws, such as those which limit the stature of man or the age to which he can attain.

But this is not so; the mortality in early life varies widely in different countries, in different parts of the same country, and in the same country at different times. Thus, while in some parts of Germany the mortality under one year was recently as high as 25 to 30 per cent. of the total births, and in England as 15, it was only a little above 10 per cent. in Norway. Infantile mortality is higher in manufacturing districts, lower in those which are agricultural, and varies from 16 per cent. in Lancashire to 9 in Dorsetshire. It is then evident that mortality in infancy is in part dependent on remediable causes; and of this there is no better proof than the fact that the mortality in England under one year has been reduced from 15 per cent. in 1872 to 13 per cent. in 1882.

It would lead us far from any practical purpose if we were to examine into all the causes which govern the liability to disease and death during infancy and childhood, in the different ranks of society. We must therefore limit our inquiry to those conditions which are met with in the class to which my readers may fairly be assumed to belong.

First among the causes of sickly infancy and premature death may be mentioned the intermarriage of near relatives. The experience of the breeders of animals, who, by what is termed breeding in and in, undoubtedly obtain certain qualities of speed, or strength, or beauty, does not apply here. They select for their experiments animals whose qualities in these respects are pre-eminent, and eliminate from them all who do not occupy the first rank. In family intermarriages, however, it is rare that any consideration is regarded, save that of wealth; and the fact remains, explain it as we may, that the intermarriage of near relatives during several successive generations is followed by a marked deterioration of the children, physical, mental, and moral; and by the intensifying of any hereditary predisposition to consumption, scrofula, and other constitutional ailments which form the second great cause of early sickness and mortality.

These are facts known to all, which yet it is not easy to represent by figures. All the world is aware that consumption is hereditary, that consumptive parents are more likely than others to have consumptive children; and a fourth of all the patients admitted into the Hospital for Consumption at Brompton stated that the disease had existed in one or other of their parents.[1] Scrofula, which is another disease closely allied to consumption, is hereditary also; and hip disease, disease of the spine, abscesses, and enlarged glands in any members of a family, point to risks for the offspring which should not be forgotten, how much soever mental endowments, personal beauty, or the charms of disposition may be considered, and sometimes reasonably enough, to outweigh them. The same liability exists with reference to epilepsy, insanity, and the whole class of affections of the nervous system. Parents inquire, with no misplaced solicitude, what is her fortune, or what are the pecuniary resources of him to whom they are asked to entrust their son's or daughter's future. Believe me, the question--what is the health of his family, or of hers? is consumption hereditary, or scrofula, or epilepsy, or insanity?--is of far greater moment, and touches much more nearly the future happiness of those we love.

These two points regard the future parents themselves; but there are other conditions on which the health of children to a great degree depends; and of these the two most important are the dwelling they inhabit, and the food they eat.

I do not refer here to the dwellings of the poor, situated in unhealthy localities, where fresh air does not enter, where the rays of the sun do not penetrate, with defective drainage and imperfect water-supply; but I speak of the nurseries of well-to-do people. 'This will do for our bedroom, and that will make a nice spare room, and that will do for the children,' is what one often hears. Had you rare plants which cost much money to obtain, which needed sunlight, warmth, and air, would you not consider anxiously the position of your conservatory, and take much pains to insure that nothing should be wanting that could help their development, so that you might feast your eyes upon their beauty, or delight yourselves with their fragrance? And yet a room at the top of the house, one of the attics perhaps, is too often destined for the little one and its nurse; or if there are two or three children, one small room is set apart for the day nursery, and a second, probably with a different aspect, for a sleeping room, and so small that it does not furnish the needed five hundred cubic feet of air for each. And as a consequence, the children are ailing, any predisposition in them to hereditary disease is fostered, they have no strength to battle against any acute illness that may befall them, and yet surprise is felt that the doctor is never out of the house.[2]

It is needless to dwell on the hand-feeding of infants as one of the great causes of mortality in infancy, and of sickliness in later life. The statistics of Foundling Hospitals bear sad testimony to the fact of its dangers, and the researches of physicians show that a peculiar form of disease is produced by it, attended by symptoms, and giving rise to appearances after death, peculiar to the form of slow starvation from which the infant has perished. I will add, because it is not generally known, one fresh illustration of the influence of artificial feeding in aggravating the mortality of infants. In Berlin the certificates of death of all infants under the age of one year, are required to state whether the little one had been brought up at the breast, or on some kind or other of artificial food. Of ten thousand children dying under the age of one year, one-fourth had been brought up at the breast, three-fourths by hand.[3]

It is, as I said in the preface, no part of my plan to enter on any details with reference to the management of children in health. It may, therefore, suffice to have pointed out the four great causes of preventible disease among the wealthier classes of society; namely, the intermarriage of near relatives, the transmission of constitutional taint, the insanitary condition of the dwelling, and the injudicious selection of the food of the infant.

FOOTNOTES:

[1] This is the proportion stated in Quain's Dictionary of Medicine, to which the writer, Dr. Theodore Williams, adds that of 1,000 cases in the upper classes 12 per cent. showed direct hereditary predisposition, and 48 per cent. family predisposition.

[2] Many useful suggestions will be found in Mrs. Gladstone's little tract, Healthy Nurseries and Bedrooms, published as one of the Health Exhibition Handbooks.

[3] The actual numbers are 2,628 and 7,646. See Generalbericht ueber das Medizinal-und Sanit 鋞 swesen der Stadt Berlin im Jahre 1881. 8vo. Berlin 1883, p. 19.

CHAPTER II.

THE GENERAL SIGNS OF DISEASE IN INFANCY AND CHILDHOOD.

The signs of disease at all ages may be referred to one or other of three great classes: disorder of function, alteration of temperature, complaint of pain.

In the infant it is the last of these which very often calls attention to the illness from which it is suffering. Cries are the only language which a young baby has to express its distress; as smiles and laughter and merry antics tell without a word its gladness. The baby must be ill, is all that its cries tell one person; another, who has seen much of sick children, will gather from them more, and will be able to judge whether its suffering is in the head, or chest, or stomach. The cries of a baby with stomach-ache are long and loud and passionate; it sheds a profusion of tears; now stops for a moment, and then begins again, drawing up its legs to its stomach; and as the pain passes off, stretches them out again, and with many little sobs passes off into a quiet sleep. If it has inflammation of the chest it does not cry aloud, it sheds no tears, but every few minutes, especially after drawing a deeper breath than before, or after each short hacking cough, it gives a little cry, which it checks apparently before it is half finished; and this, either because it has no breath to waste in cries, or because the effort makes its breathing more painful. If disease is going on in the head, the child utters sharp piercing shrieks, and then between whiles a low moan or wail, or perhaps no sound at all, but lies quiet, apparently dozing, till pain wakes it up again.

It is not, however, by the cry alone, or by any one sign of disease, that it is possible to judge either of its nature or of its degree, but the mention of this serves merely as an illustration, which anyone can understand, of the different meanings that even a baby's cry will convey to different persons.

When a child is taken ill, be the disease from which it is about to suffer what it may, there is at once a change from its condition when in health, such as soon attracts the attention even of the least observant. The child loses its appetite, is fretful and soon tired, and either very sleepy or very restless, while most likely it is thirsty, and its skin hotter than natural. In many instances, too, it feels sick or actually vomits, while its bowels are either much purged or very bound. If old enough to talk, it generally complains of feeling ill, or says that it has pain in some part or other, though it is by no means certain that a little child has described rightly the seat of its pain; for it very often says that its head aches or that its stomach aches, just because it has heard people when ill complain of pain in the head or in the stomach. Some of these signs of illness are, of course, absent in the infant, who can describe its feelings even by signs imperfectly; but the baby loses its merry laugh and its cheerful look; it ceases to watch its mother's or its nurse's eye as it was used to do, though it clings to her more closely than ever, and will not be out of her arms even for a moment; and if at length rocked to sleep in her lap, will yet wake up and cry immediately on being placed in its cot again.

Symptoms such as these are sure to awaken the mother's attention to her child, and the child's welfare and the parent's happiness alike depend, in many instances, on the way in which she sets about to answer the question, 'What is the matter?'

Some mothers send at once to the doctor whenever they see or fancy that anything ails their child. But this way of getting rid of responsibility is not always possible, nor, indeed, on moral grounds, is it always desirable, for the mother who delegates each unpleasant duty to another, whether nurse, governess, or doctor, in order to save herself trouble or anxiety, performs but half a mother's part, and can expect but half a mother's recompense of love.

Whenever a child is unwell, a mother may do much to ascertain what is the matter, and may by the exercise of a little patience and common sense save herself much needless heart-ache, and her child much suffering.

The first point to ascertain is the presence or absence of fever; that is to say, whether, and how much, the temperature of the body is higher than natural. If the temperature is not higher than natural, it may be taken as almost certain that the child neither has any inflammatory affection of the chest, nor is about to suffer from any of the eruptive fevers. The temperature, however, cannot be judged of merely by the sensation conveyed to the hand, but must be ascertained by means of the thermometer.[4] In the case of the grown person the thermometer is placed either under the tongue, the lips being closed over it, or in the armpit, and is kept there five or six minutes. In young children, however, neither of these is practicable, and I prefer to place the instrument in the groin, and crossing one leg over the other, to maintain the thermometer there for the requisite five minutes. The temperature of the body in health is about 98.5?Fahr. in the grown person, and very slightly higher in childhood; but any heat above 99.5?may be regarded as evidence that something is wrong, and the persistence for more than twenty-four hours of a temperature of 101?and upwards, may be taken as almost conclusive proof of the existence of some serious inflammation, or of the onset of one of the eruptive fevers.

At the same time it is well to bear in mind that temporary causes, such as especially the disorders produced by over-fatigue, or by an over-hearty or indigestible meal, may suddenly raise the temperature as high as 102? or higher, but the needed repose or the action of a purgative may be followed in a few hours by an almost equally sudden decline of the heat to the natural standard.

It is well to learn to count the pulse and the frequency of the breathing; but to do the former accurately, requires practice such as is hardly gained except by hospital training; and indeed, with few exceptions, the value of the information furnished by the pulse is less in the child than in the adult. The reasons for this are obvious, since the rapidity of the circulation varies under the slightest causes, and the very constraint of holding the sick child's hand makes it struggle, and its efforts raise the frequency of the heart-beats by ten or twenty in the minute. The place at which to seek the beat of the pulse is at the wrist, just inside and below the protuberance of the wrist-bone; but if the child is very fat it is often difficult to detect it. When detected it is not easy to count it in early infancy, for during the first year of life the heart beats between 120 and 130 in the minute, diminishing between that age and five years to 100, and gradually sinking to 90 at twelve years old. In proportion, moreover, to the tender age of the child, is the rapidity of its circulation apt to vary under the influence of slight causes, while both its frequency and that of the breathing are about a third less during sleep than in the waking state.

The frequency of the breathing is less difficult to ascertain, while at the same time it furnishes more reliable information than the pulse. This is best tested when the child is asleep, remembering always that the breathing is then slower than in the waking state. The open hand, well warmed, should be laid flat and gently over the child's night-dress on the lower part of the chest and the pit of the stomach. Each heaving of the chest, which marks a fresh breath being taken, may be counted, and the information thus obtained is very valuable. Up to the age of two years the child breathes from 30 to 40 times in a minute, and this frequency gradually declines to from 25 to 30 till the age of twelve, and then settles down to from 20 to 25 as in the grown person. You would thus know that a sleeping infant who was breathing more than 30 times, or a child of five who breathes more than 25 times, has some ailment in its chest, and that the doctor should be sent for in order to ascertain its exact nature.

It would answer no good purpose to give a description of the information to be obtained by listening to the chest. To learn from this, needs the well-trained ear; and harm, not good, comes from the half-knowledge which serves but to lead astray.

A child may be very suffering, seem very ill, and its suffering and illness may depend on pain in the stomach owing to indigestion, constipation, or even to an accidental chill. After early infancy it is not difficult to make out the seat of the child's suffering: the warm hand placed gently on its stomach will soon ascertain whether it is tense or tender, whether the tenderness is confined to one particular spot, or whether it is more acute at one spot than at another; and, lastly, whether, as is the case when pain is produced by wind in the intestines, the pain and tenderness are both relieved by gentle rubbing.

In the young infant the character of the cry will, as I have already said, give some clue to the seat of its pain, while, if you lay it down in its cot or in its nurse's arms in order to examine its stomach, it will often resist and begin to cry. Its stomach then becomes perfectly tense, and you cannot tell whether pressure on it causes pain or whether the cries are not altogether the consequence of fretfulness and fear. It is therefore the best plan to pass your hand beneath the child's clothes and to examine its stomach without altering its posture, while at the same time the nurse in whose arms it is talks to it to distract its attention, or holds it opposite the window, or opposite a bright light, which seldom fails to amuse an infant. If there is no tenderness of the stomach the child will not cry on pressure; or if during your examination the presence of wind in the intestines should occasion pain, gentle friction, instead of increasing suffering, will give relief.

The one thing which still remains to do, especially in the case of children in whom teething is not over, is to examine the mouth and ascertain the state of the gums, since some ailments are caused and others are aggravated by teething. A wise mother or an intelligent nurse will teach the child when well the little trick of putting out its tongue and opening its mouth to show its teeth when told to do so; and though it may sometimes indulge rather out of place in these performances when wished to behave especially prettily before strangers, yet when older it will quickly learn the proprieties of behaviour, and in the meanwhile you profit much by the lesson when illness really comes.

Sometimes, however, infants who when well will open their mouth and allow their gums to be felt without difficulty, refuse to do so when ill; and it is always desirable that the mother or nurse whose duty it is to tend the sick child constantly, should not frighten it, or lose its confidence, by doing forcibly that which the doctor who comes occasionally may yet be quite right in doing. You will, however, generally get a good view of the mouth and throat in young infants by gently touching the lips with your finger: the child opens its mouth instinctively, and then you can run your finger quickly over its tongue, and drawing it slightly forward perfectly see the condition of the throat, feel the gums as you withdraw your finger, and notice the appearance of the tongue. Sometimes it is important to ascertain whether a tooth which was near coming through has actually pierced the gum, and yet the child's fretfulness renders it almost impossible to induce it to open its mouth. If now, while the nurse holds the child in her arms, you go behind her, you can, unseen and unawares, introduce your finger into its mouth and ascertain all you wish to know before the little one has recovered from its surprise.

I have but little to say here about the general signs of brain disease in infancy and childhood, because they will need minute notice afterwards. All that I would at present observe is, that you must not at once conclude that a child's head is seriously affected, because it is heavy and fretful and passionate, and refuses to be amused. The head, as we know by our own experience, suffers by sympathy in the course of almost every ailment, certainly of every acute ailment, at all ages. If the babe is not sick; if its bowels can be acted on by ordinary means; if, though drowsy, it can be roused without difficulty; if, though it may prefer a darkened room, it does not shrink from the light when admitted gradually; if it has no slight twitchings of its fingers or of its wrists; if the head, though hot, is not hotter than the rest of the body; if the large vessels of the neck, or the open part of the head, or fontanelle as it is termed, in an infant in whom the head is not yet closed, are not beating violently; and, above all, if when it cries it sheds tears, you may quiet your mind on the score of the child's brain, at any rate until the doctor's visit, and may turn a deaf ear to the nurse or the friend who assures you that the child is about to have convulsions or to be attacked by inflammation of the brain.

FOOTNOTES:

[4] The thermometer used for this purpose, called a clinical thermometer, may be bought for about twelve shillings, of any chemist or instrument-maker, and its mode of employment can be learned in five minutes. No mother should be without it.

CHAPTER III.

THE GENERAL MANAGEMENT OF DISEASE IN INFANCY AND CHILDHOOD.

The management of the child when ill is difficult or easy in exact proportion to whether it has been ill or well managed when in health. The mother who lives but little with her children, who contents herself with a daily visit to the nursery, and who then scarcely sees her little ones until they are brought into the drawing-room in the evening in full dress, to be petted and admired and fondled by the visitors, cannot expect to take her place by the child's bed in its sickness, to soothe its pain, and to expend upon it all the pent-up tenderness which, in spite of the calls of business or of pleasure, still dwells within her heart. She must be content to see the infant turn from her to the nurse with whose face it has all its life been familiar; or to hear the little one tell her to go away, for her presence is associated with none of those 'familiar acts, made beautiful by love,' which win the young heart: the mother is but a stranger who brings no help, who relieves no distress. Happy such a mother if she has found a conscientious and intelligent nurse to whom she can delegate her office; but she must remember that with the child, love follows in the steps of daily, hourly kindnesses, that a mother's part must be played in health if it is to be undertaken in sickness, that it cannot be laid down and taken up again at pleasure.

There is another mother who cannot nurse her child to any good purpose, she who when it was well spoilt it from excess of love, who has yielded to each wayward wish, and has allowed it to become the petty tyrant of the household. The child is ill, it is languid, feverish, and in pain; no position is quite easy to it, no food pleasant to it, bed is irksome, medicine is nasty. It knows only that it suffers, it has been accustomed to have its will obeyed in everything, and cannot understand that its suffering is not at once taken away. It insists on getting up and on being dressed, or on lying in its mother's or nurse's lap, where the warmth of another person's body does but aggravate its fever; it screams with passion at the approach of the doctor, it will not allow itself to be examined, it will take no medicine; the doctor is powerless, the mother heart-broken. Sickness is not the time to exercise authority which has not been put in force before; and, not once but many times, I have watched, a sad spectator, the death of children from an illness not necessarily fatal, but rendered so because it was impossible to learn the progress of disease, impossible to administer the necessary remedies.

What a child has been made when well, such it will be when sick.

One more point I must insist on before going into details, and that is as to the necessity of perfect truthfulness in dealing with sick children. The foolish device of telling a child when ill, that the doctor who has been sent for is its uncle or its cousin, is the outcome of the still more foolish falsehood of threatening the child with the doctor's visit if it does not do this or that. No endeavour should be spared by nurse or parent, or by the doctor himself, to render his visit popular in the nursery. Three-fourths of the difficulties which attend the administration of medicine are commonly the result of previous bad management of the child, of foolish over-indulgence, or of still more foolish want of truthfulness. It may answer once to tell a child that medicine is nice when really it is nasty, but the trick will scarcely succeed a second time, and the one success will increase your difficulties ever after. If medicine is absolutely necessary, and the child is too young to understand reason, it must be given by force, very firmly but very kindly, and the grief it occasions will be forgotten in an hour or two. If he is old enough, tell him that the medicine is ordered to do him good, and firmness combined with gentleness will usually succeed in inducing him to take it. The advantage of perfect truthfulness extends to every incident in the illness of children, even to the not saying, 'Oh, you will soon be well,' if it is not likely so to be. If children find you never deceive them, how implicitly they will trust you, what an infinity of trouble is saved, and how much rest of mind is secured to the poor little sufferer!

A little boy three years old was ordered to be cupped. The cupper, a kind old man, said to encourage him, 'Oh, dear little boy, it's nothing.' The child turned to his mother, saying, 'Mummy, is that true?' His mother said it was not, but that for her sake she hoped he would try to bear it well. And the operation was performed without a cry or a sound.

I have spoken of the moral conditions implied in the successful management of sick children. There are certain physical conditions no less important. The sick child should not be left in the common nursery, of which he would taint the air, while he would be disturbed by its other little inmates. He must (and of course I am speaking not of some slight ailment, but of a more serious indisposition) be in a room by himself, which should be kept quiet and shaded, and at a temperature which should not be allowed to fall below 60?if the chest is in any way affected, nor to exceed 55?in other cases, and this temperature should always be measured, not by guess, but by the thermometer hung close to the child's bed. The room is to be shaded, not by curtains round the bed--for, save in special circumstances, curtains should be banished from the nursery--nor by closed shutters which exclude both light and air, but by letting down the blinds, so as to have a sort of twilight in the room, and by shading any light which at night may be burned in the apartment; while whether by day or night the child should be so placed that his face shall be turned from the light, not directed towards it. The room should be kept quiet, and this requires not only general quiet in the house, but quiet in the movements of all persons in the room; speaking, not in a whisper, but in a low and gentle voice; walking carefully, not in a silk dress nor in creaky shoes, but not on tiptoe, for there is a fussy sham quietness which disturbs the sick far more than the loudest noise.

Little precautions, so trifling that few think of noticing them, have much to do with the quiet of the sick-room, and consequently with the patient's comfort. A rattling window will keep a child awake for hours, or the creaking handle of the door rouse it up again each time anyone enters the room; and to put a wedge in the window, or to tie back the handle, and so quietly open and close the door, may do more than medicine towards promoting the child's recovery. There can, however, be no abiding quiet without a well-ordered room, and the old proverb carried out, 'A place for everything, and everything in its place.' A table covered with a cloth so that things may be taken up and put down noiselessly, and set apart for the medicine, the drink, the nourishment, cups, glasses, spoons, or whatever else the patient is in frequent need of; with a wooden bowl and water for rinsing cups and glasses in, and a cloth or two for wiping them, will save much trouble and noise, and the loud whispers of the attendants to each other, 'Where is the sugar? where is the arrowroot? where did you put down the medicine?' of which we hear so much in the sick-room, so much especially in the sick-room of the child, who is unable to tell how extremely all this disturbs him.

One more caution still remains for me to give. Do not talk to the doctor in the child's room, do not relate bad symptoms, do not express your fears, nor ask the doctor his opinion in the child's hearing. The child often understands much more than you would imagine, misunderstands still more; and over and over again I have known the thoughtless utterance of the mother, nurse, or doctor depress a child's spirits and seriously retard his recovery.

It is consoling to bear in mind that how grave soever a child's illness may be, the power of repair is greater in early life than in adult age, that with few exceptions the probability of recovery is greater in the child than it would be from the same disease in the grown person. This too is due not simply to the activity of the reparative powers in early life, but also in great measure to the mental and moral characteristics of childhood.

To make the sick child happy, in order that he may get well, is the unwritten lesson which they who have best learnt, know best how to nurse sick children. It may seem strange, that from so high a purpose I should at once come down to so commonplace a detail as to insist on the importance, even on this account, of keeping the sick child in bed.

At the onset of every illness of which the nature is not obvious, during the course of any illness in which the chest is affected, or in which the temperature is higher than natural, bed is the best and happiest place for the child. In it repose is most complete, far more complete than after early babyhood it can be in the nurse's or mother's lap, and free from the great objection of the increased heat from being in contact with another person's body. Nothing is more painful than to witness the little child, sick and feverish, with heavy eyes, and aching head, up and dressed, trying to amuse itself with its customary toys; then, with 'Please nurse me,' begging to be taken in the lap, then getting down again; fretful, and sad, and passionate by turns; dragging about its misery, wearing out its little strength, in deference to the prejudice that bed is so weakening.

The bed does not weaken, but the disease does which renders bed necessary.

A child frets sometimes at the commencement of an illness if kept in its own little cot. But put it in its nurse's or mother's big bed, set a tea tray with some new toys upon it before the child, and a pillow behind it, so that when tired with play it may lie back and go to sleep, and you will have husbanded its strength and saved your own, have halved your anxiety and doubled the child's happiness.

Young infants, indeed, when ill often refuse to be put out of the arms, but over and over again I have found the experiment succeed of laying the baby on a bed, the nurse or mother lying down by its side, and soothing it to sleep. Were there no other drawback, it is a waste of power to have two persons employed in nursing a sick child; one to keep it in her lap, and the other to wait upon her.

It is important in all serious illnesses of children, as well as of a grown person, that the bed should be so placed that the attendant can pass on either side, and can from either side reach the patient to do whatever is necessary. Most cots for young children have a rail round them to prevent the child falling out of bed when asleep or at play; but nothing can be more inconvenient than the fixed rail over which the attendant has to bend in order to give the child food or medicine, or for any other purpose. When I founded the Children's Hospital in Ormond Street, I introduced children's cots (the idea of which I took from those in the Children's Hospital at Frankfort) the sides of which let down when needed, while on the top of the rail, or dependent from it, a board is placed surrounded by a raised beading on which the toys, the food, or drink may be put with great convenience. These bedsteads, with probably some improved arrangement for letting down the sides, may be seen now in most children's hospitals, but I have been surprised to observe how seldom they are employed in private nurseries, and how comparatively few bedstead-makers are acquainted with them. The result would probably have been very different had a patent been taken out for them, and had they been largely advertised as 'Dr. West's improved children's bedsteads'! The uninclosed spring mattress, and the wedge-shaped horsehair cushion, both of which I introduced in Ormond Street, are also very valuable. The latter slightly raises the head and shoulders, and renders any other than a thin horsehair pillow for the head to rest on unnecessary.

A few more hints about the bed may not be out of place. First of all, after early infancy is over, at latest after nine months, except for some very special reason the napkin should be done away with. It heats the child, chafes it, and makes it sore; it conceals the inattention of the nurse, and at the same time renders it less easy to keep the little one absolutely clean than if a folded napkin is placed under the hips, whence it can be at once removed when soiled. In all serious illness a piece of macintosh should be placed under the sheet, as is done in the lying-in room, and a draw-sheet, as it is termed, over it. The draw-sheet is, as its name implies, a folded sheet, laid under the hips, and withdrawn in part when needed so as to prevent the child ever lying on linen that is wet or soiled. It can be drawn away from under the child, and a portion still clean and dry brought under it, while the soiled part is rolled together and wrapped up in macintosh at one side of the bed until a new draw sheet is substituted, which is easily done by tacking a fresh sheet to that which is about to be withdrawn, when the fresh one is brought under the child's body as that which is soiled is removed. The greatest care should always be taken that the under sheet is perfectly free from ruck or wrinkle; in long illnesses the skin becomes chafed and bed-sores may be produced by neglect of this simple precaution. The complaint that a child throws off the bed-clothes is easily remedied by a couple of bits of tape tied on either side loosely from the sheet or blanket to the sides of the cot.

When children are compelled to remain long in bed, great care is needed to prevent the skin from being chafed, which is the first step that leads to the occurrence of bed-sores. Careful washing with soap and water daily of the whole body, not only of those parts which may be soiled by the urine or the evacuations; the washing afterwards with pure tepid water; careful drying, and abundant powdering with starch powder, will do much to prevent the accident. If, in spite of this care, the skin seems anywhere to be red or chafed, it should be sponged over with brandy or with sweet spirits of nitre before powdering. Real bed-sores must be seen and treated by the doctor.

The warm bath is a great source of comfort to the sick child, and in all cases of feverishness, of influenza, or threatening bronchitis, it should not be omitted before the child is put to bed, or must be given towards evening if the child has not been up during the day. The bath may be either warm or hot, the temperature of the former being 90?to 92? that of the latter 95?to 96? The temperature should always be ascertained by the thermometer, and the warm bath only should be employed, except when the hot bath is ordered by the doctor. The warm bath relieves feverishness and quiets the system, and promotes gentle perspiration; the hot bath is given when the eruption of scarlet fever or of measles fails to come out properly, or in some cases of convulsions at the same time that cold is applied to the head, or, in some forms of dropsy when it is of importance to excite the action of the skin as much as possible. It is not desirable that a child should remain less than five or more than ten minutes in the bath, and attention must be paid by the addition of warm water to maintain the bath at the same temperature during the whole time of the child's immersion.

Now and then infants and very young children when ill seem frightened at the bath, and then instead of being soothed and relieved by it they are only excited and distressed. If the bath is brought into the room, prepared in the child's sight, and he is then taken out of bed, undressed, and put into the water which he sees steaming before him, he very often becomes greatly alarmed, struggles violently, cries passionately, and does not become quiet again till he has sobbed himself to sleep. All this time, however, he has been exerting his inflamed lungs to the utmost, and will probably have thereby done himself ten times more harm than the bath has done good. Very different would it have been if the bath had been got ready out of the child's sight; if when brought to the bedside it had been covered with a blanket so as to hide the steam; if the child had been laid upon the blanket, and gently let down into the water, and this even without undressing him if he were very fearful; and then if you wish to make a baby quite happy in the water, put in a couple of bungs or corks with feathers stuck in them, for the baby to play with. Managed thus, I have often seen the much-dreaded bath become a real delight to the little one, and have found that if tears were shed at all, it was at being taken out of the water, not at being placed in it.

In a great variety of conditions, poultices are of use. They are needed in the case of abscesses which it is wished to bring to a head; they are sometimes applied over wounds which are in an unhealthy condition, or from which it is desired to keep up a discharge. They soothe the pain of stomach-ache from any cause, and are of most essential service when constantly applied in many forms of chest inflammation. And yet not one mother or nurse in ten knows how to make a poultice.[5] When applied over a wound they should not be covered with oiled silk or any impermeable material, since the edges of the wound and the adjacent skin are apt thereby to be rendered irritable and to become covered with little itching pimples. When used to relieve pain in the stomach, or as a warm application in cases of inflammation of the chest, they should be covered with some impermeable material, and will then not require to be changed oftener than every six hours. After poultices have been applied over the chest or stomach for two or three days the skin is apt to become tender, and then it is well to substitute for them what may be termed a dry poultice, which is nothing else than a layer of dry cotton wool an inch or an inch and a half thick, tacked inside a piece of oiled silk.

A handy substitute for a poultice may be made of bran stitched in a flannel bag, heated by pouring boiling water on it, then squeezed as dry as possible and laid over the painful part. This is especially useful to relieve the stomach-ache of infants and young children.

Spongio-piline is a useful substitute for a poultice, especially when it is desirable to employ a soothing or stimulating liniment to the surface. It retains heat very well when wrung out of hot water, and any liniment sprinkled on it is brought into contact with the skin much better than if diffused through a poultice. I may just add that its edges should be sloped inwards, in order to prevent the moisture from it oozing out and wetting the child's night-dress.

When I was young, leeches and bleeding were frequently, no doubt too frequently, employed. We have now, however, gone too much to the other extreme, for cases are met with from time to time of congestion of the brain, or of inflammation of the chest or of the bowels, in which leeches bring greater and more speedy relief than any other remedy. In applying leeches it is always desirable that they should be put on where they will be out of the child's sight if possible, and where it will be comparatively easy to stop the bleeding. Hence, in many instances of inflammation of the bowels, it is better to apply the leeches at the edge of the lower bowel, the anus as it is technically termed, than on the front of the stomach, though, of course, this will not always answer the purpose. Leeches to the chest may usually be put on just under the shoulder-blade; and leeches to the head on one or other side behind the ear, where they will be out of the way of any large vein, and where the pressure of the finger will easily stop the bleeding. Steady pressure with the finger will, even where there is no bone to press against, usually effect this; and then a little pad of lint put over the bite, and one or two layers over that, and all fastened on with strips of adhesive plaster, will prevent any renewal of the bleeding. In the few cases where it is not arrested by these means, the application of a little of the solution of muriate of iron will hardly fail of effect.

There is one more point to which I will refer before passing lastly to the question of how to manage in the administration of medicine; and this is the best way of applying cold to the head. This is often ordered, but very seldom efficiently done. Cold is best applied by means of a couple of bladders half-filled with pounded ice, and wrapped in two large napkins; one of them should be placed under the child's head, the corners of the napkin being pinned to the pillow-case to prevent its being disturbed, while the other is allowed to rest upon the head, but with the corners of the napkin again pinned to the pillow so as to take off the greater part of its weight. Thus arranged, the cold application will neither get displaced by the child's movements, nor will the child itself be wetted, as it too commonly is when wet cloths are employed for this purpose, nor irritated by their perpetual removal and renewal.

In London and in large towns there are various contrivances of vulcanised rubber, which are, of course, far preferable to the bladders, but it is not everyone who lives in London, or who can command the resources furnished by a large city.

The difficulties in the administration of medicine to children are in great part the fault, either of the doctor in giving needlessly unpleasant medicine, or of the parents or nurse who either have failed to teach the child obedience, or who are deficient in that tact by which hundreds of small troubles are evaded.

As far as the doctor is concerned, all medicines should be prescribed by him in small quantities, and as free from taste and smell as possible: or where that cannot be, the unpleasant flavour should be covered by syrup, or liquorice, or treacle.

Bulky powders should be avoided, and the child who has learned to take rhubarb and magnesia, or Gregory's powder without resistance, certainly does credit to his training.

Aperients are the medicines most frequently needed in the minor ailments of children, and a wise mother will not undertake herself the management of serious diseases. Of all aperients castor oil is perhaps the safest, the least irritating, the most generally applicable; it acts on the bowels and does nothing more. The idea that it tends specially to produce constipation afterwards is unfounded; it does not do so more than other aperients. All aperients quicken for a time what is termed the peristaltic action of the bowels; that is to say, their constant movement in a direction from the stomach to the lower bowel, which, as well as a contraction on themselves, is constantly going on in every living animal, and continues even for some time after death. The bowels stimulated to greater activity of movement by the aperient, become for a time more sluggish afterwards; they rest for a while, just as after a long walk the muscles of the leg are weary and need repose.

There are indeed aperients which do more than this, as grey powder and calomel act upon the liver, and so by promoting an increased flow of bile cause a more permanent excitement of the bowels, and consequently their more prolonged activity; or as Epsom salts or citrate of magnesia, which by their action on the blood cause a greater secretion or pouring out of fluid from the coats of the intestines, and in this way have in addition to their purgative property a special influence in abating various feverish conditions.

Castor oil, senna, jalap, jalapine, and scammony are simple aperients. They empty the bowels and nothing more, and in cases of simple constipation, or where a child is ill either from eating too much or from taking indigestible food, are the best purgatives that can be given. A dose of castor oil, often one of the great griefs of the nursery, may generally be given without the least difficulty if previously shaken up in a bottle with a wine-glassful of hot milk sweetened and flavoured with a piece of cinnamon boiled in it, by which all taste of the oil is effectually concealed.

The domestic remedy, senna tea with prunes which render it palatable, confection of senna, syrup of senna, and the sweet essence of senna are generally very readily taken by children, but all have the disadvantage of being liable to gripe. The German liquorice powder, as it is called, which is composed of powdered senna, liquorice powder, fennel, and a little sulphur with white sugar, is freer from this drawback than any other preparation, and when mixed with a little water is not generally objected to. It is important, as senna is often adulterated and loses its properties by exposure to the air, that this powder should always be obtained from a very good chemist, purchased in small quantities, and always kept in a glass-stoppered bottle.

Jalap, in the form in which it is usually sold--as compound jalap powder--is in general readily taken; it acts speedily, but often with pain, and is not a desirable domestic remedy. Jalapine, which is a sort of extract of jalap, is much less apt to gripe, and owing to its small bulk is much handier. It may be given in doses of from two to five grains to children from two years old and upwards.

Scammony is another powerful simple aperient, apt to be violent in its action, and therefore not to be given except when the bowels have long been confined, or when it is given to expel worms. The compound scammony powder is the form in which it is usually given, and of that five grains would be a dose for a child two years old.

Scammony, however, is a costly drug, and therefore the caution given with reference to German liquorice powder applies here also.

There is a preparation of scammony, the so-called scammony mixture, which consists of the resin or extract of scammony dissolved in milk, which is extremely useful when the stomach is irritable, or there is much difficulty in inducing the child to take medicine. It is almost tasteless, and a tablespoonful, which would be a proper dose for a child of five years old, can be given without being detected.

Much of the difficulty experienced in giving powders arises from their being mixed with the arrowroot or jam in which they are administered. A very small quantity of arrowroot, bread and milk, or jam, should be put in a tea-spoon; the powder then laid upon it, and covered over with the arrowroot or jelly, so, in short, as to make a kind of sandwich, with the powder, which would thus be untasted, in the middle.

Aloes is a purgative which acts chiefly on the large bowel and to some degree also on the liver, and is of most use in the habitual constipation of weakly children. In spite of its bitter taste the powder is seldom objected to if given between two layers of coarse brown sugar, while with most children the addition of a teaspoonful of treacle will induce them to take very readily that useful medicine, the compound decoction of aloes.

Both rhubarb, aloes, and indeed other remedies which are nauseous if given as a liquid and are bulky in the form of powder, may very readily be given in extract in the form of very tiny pills. Thus I have constantly ordered the extract of rhubarb, which is nearly twice as strong as the powder, made up into pills scarcely bigger than what children call 'hundreds and thousands' and silver-coated. Ten or a dozen of these go down in a teaspoonful of jelly unknown, and with no expenditure of temper or tears.

The citrate of magnesia, or Dinneford's Magnesia, taken effervescing with lemon juice, or when the effervescence has passed off, or the French Limonade Purgative, are almost always very readily taken, and are often very useful in the little febrile attacks, or in the slight feverish rashes to which children are liable in the spring and autumn.

Mercurials should have no place among domestic remedies. I do not mean that the doctor need be called in to prescribe each time that they are given, but that the mother should learn from him distinctly with reference to each individual child the circumstances which justify their employment. They stimulate the liver, as well as produce thereby action of the bowels, but they have, especially if often employed, a far-reaching influence on the constitution, and that undoubtedly of a depressing kind: an influence more than made up for when really needed by their other qualities, and especially by their power in doing away with the results of many forms of chronic inflammation. They are 'edged tools,' however, and we know the proverb about those who play with them.[6]

Grey powder, blue pill, and calomel are the three forms in one or other of which mercurials are commonly given. Of the three, grey powder is the mildest; but it has the inconvenience of not infrequently causing nausea, or actual sickness. This objection does not apply to blue pill, which can be given either in the tiny pills of which I have already spoken, or else broken down, and given in a little jam, or in a teaspoonful of syrup or treacle. On the whole I prefer calomel in small doses. It has the great advantage of tastelessness, small bulk, and of never causing sickness. Half a grain of calomel may be regarded as equivalent to two grains of grey powder or blue pill.

I shall speak afterwards of other medicines, which may in various circumstances be given, to act upon the bowels; but the above include all that are at all fit for common use in the nursery.

Before leaving this subject I will add a word or two about the use of suppositories and lavements in infancy and childhood. A piece of paper rolled up into a conical form and greased, or a bit of soap, is not infrequently introduced by nurses just within the bowel, as a means of overcoming constipation in infants. The irritation of the muscle at its orifice (the sphincter, as it is termed) excites the bowels to action, and does away with the necessity for giving an aperient. The drawback from this, as well as from the use of the lavement, is that if frequently employed they become habitually necessary, and the bowels will then never act without their customary stimulus. The lavement, too, has the additional disadvantage that while the lower part of the bowel is in proportion more capacious in infancy and childhood than in the adult, this peculiarity becomes exaggerated by the constant distension of the intestine, and a larger and still larger quantity of fluid needs to be thrown up in order to produce the requisite action of the bowels.

Opiates and other soothing medicines should never be given except when prescribed by the doctor. Thirty-two deaths in England under five years of age in 1882 represent but a very small part of the evil wrought by the overdose or injudicious use of these remedies. Above all, soothing medicines of varying strength, as syrup of poppies, or of unknown composition, as Dalby's Carminative or Winslow's Soothing Syrup, should never be employed. The only safe preparation, and this to be given only by the doctor's orders or with his approval, is the compound tincture of camphor, or paregoric elixir, as it is called, of which sixty measured drops contain a quarter of a grain of opium. Ten to fifteen measured drops of this are a sufficient dose for a child one year old, and this ought not to be repeated within twelve hours. The repetition every few hours of small doses of opiates is quite as hazardous as the giving of a single overdose; and if it does not work serious mischief by stupefying the child, it renders it impossible to judge of its real condition.

Thus much may suffice with reference to the more important remedies. Others will necessarily call for notice when the diseases come to be considered in which they may be of service.

There are two points which still remain to be noticed before I leave the introductory part of this little book.

The first of these concerns the importance of keeping written notes in the course of every case of serious illness. For want of doing this the most imperfect and conflicting accounts of what has happened are given to the doctor. No person can watch to any good purpose for four-and-twenty hours together; and no one's memory, least of all in the midst of fatigue and anxiety, can correctly retain all details concerning medicine, food, and sleep, which yet it may be of paramount importance that the doctor should be made acquainted with. I am accustomed to desire a record to be kept on a sheet of paper divided into six columns, one for food, a second for medicine, a third for sleep, a fourth for the evacuations, and a fifth for any special point which the nature of the illness renders it of special moment to observe, while the date is entered on the first column of all, indicating when food or medicine was given, or when and for how long the child slept. It is best to enter the variations of temperature on a separate paper, in order that the doctor may at a glance perceive the daily changes in this important respect. No one who has not made the experiment can tell the relief which the keeping this simple record gives to the anxiety of nursing the sick, especially when the sick one is loved most tenderly.

The other point concerns the relations of the mother or of the parents to the doctor. I have often heard it said, 'Dr. Green always attends my husband and myself, but we have Dr. White for the servants and children,' implying a lower degree of medical knowledge as required in their case, and to be acknowledged by a lower rate of remuneration.

Need I say that the assumption is a mistaken one--that as much knowledge, as large experience, are needed in the one case as in the other; while over and above, to treat children successfully, a special tact and a special fondness for children are needed? A man may be a very good doctor without those special gifts; but their possession, apart from real medical knowledge, may make a good children's nurse, but never a good children's doctor.

Another matter not to be forgotten is the confidence to be reposed in the doctor--the readiness to acquiesce in his sometimes visiting the child more frequently in the course of an illness than the symptoms may seem to you to require. Were you involved in some civil action, in which your succession to large property was involved, you would scarcely expect your solicitor to give you his opinion on all the questions at a single interview. In the same way, the doctor, even the most experienced, may need to visit his little patient several times before he can feel quite certain as to the nature of the disease that is impending, while he may not wish to alarm you by suggesting all the possibilities that are present to his mind. The child after a restless night may be asleep, and it may be most undesirable to wake him; or he may be excessively cross and unmanageable, so that it is impossible to listen to his chest; or it may be very important to ascertain whether the high temperature present in the morning has risen still higher towards night, or whether, after free action of the bowels, it has fallen a degree or two, showing that no fever is impending, but that the undue heat of the body was occasioned by the constipation. Or, again, some remedy may have been ordered, of the effect of which the doctor does not feel quite sure: he wishes to see for himself whether it is right to continue or wiser to suspend it. The wise physician, like the able general, leaves as little as may be to chance.

Nearly forty years ago, in addressing a class of medical students, I said to them:

'If you are carefully to observe all the points which I have mentioned, and to make yourselves thoroughly masters of a case, you must be lavish of your time; you must be content to turn aside from the direct course of investigation, which you would pursue uninterruptedly in the adult, in order to soothe the waywardness of the child, to quiet its fears, or even to cheat it into good humour by joining in its play; and you must be ready to do this, not the first time only, but every time that you visit the child, and must try to win its affections in order to cure its disease. If you fail in the former, you will often be foiled in your attempts at the latter. Nor is this all; you must visit your patient very often if the disease is serious in its nature and rapid in its course. New symptoms succeed each other in infancy and childhood with great rapidity; complications occur that call for some change in your treatment, or the vital powers falter suddenly when you least expect it. The issues of life and death often hang on the immediate adoption of a certain plan of treatment, or on its timely discontinuance. Do not wait, therefore, for symptoms of great urgency before you visit a child three or four times a day; but if the disease is one in which changes are likely to take place rapidly, be frequent in your visits as well as watchful in your observation.'

Each year has added to my conviction of the perfect truth of each word which I have quoted. If you believe your doctor to be a man of integrity and intelligence, be thankful for his frequent visits, which will cease as his anxiety abates. Be convinced that in the mean time they are made, not for his sake, but for yours. If you doubt his integrity, change your doctor; but do not say to him in a tone and with an emphasis which there is no mistaking, 'Well, if you think it really necessary to come'!

FOOTNOTES:

[5] I add in this note a few simple directions for making poultices, though, as I have stated in my preface, it is no part of my purpose to enter into all the details, important though they are, of a sick nurse's duties.

For a linseed meal poultice, see that the water is boiling, not merely hot; warm the basin, put the water in first; sprinkle the meal on it, stirring the whole time, till it becomes of the uniform consistency of porridge, then spread it about half an inch thick over the linen, or whatever it is spread on, and turn up the edges for an inch all round to prevent the poultice crumbling and soiling the night-dress; and then having smeared the surface with a little oil, test its warmth by applying it to your cheek before putting it on the patient. A broad bandage of some sort or a soft towel must then be put round the body to keep the poultice in its place, and secured with safety pins.

Pure mustard poultices are never used in children, on account of the pain they occasion, and the too great irritation which they would cause of the delicate skin of children. A mixture of one part of mustard to two of linseed meal is, however, often of much use in the chest affections of children.

Bread poultices are less generally useful than those of linseed meal. They do not retain the heat nearly so well as those of linseed meal, and are chiefly used in cuts, wounds, or small abscesses; and also because they are so easily made. A slice of stale bread without the crust is put on a plate, boiling water is poured over it, and drained off; it is then placed on a piece of muslin, pressed between two plates to squeeze out the remaining water, and its surface is greased before it is applied with a little oil or lard. I would refer for details about how to make poultices, and for many other things well worth the knowing, to Miss Wood's Handbook of Nursing, London, 12mo, 1883.

[6] I am not ignorant of the doubts which have been raised with reference to the special influence of mercurial remedies on the liver, but prefer in a book written for non-medical readers to leave the popular opinion unquestioned.

PART II.

All that has been said hitherto is only introductory to the great purpose of this book, which is to give an account of the nature, symptoms, and course of the more important diseases of infancy and childhood.

Any attempt at scientific arrangement of a popular book is useless. I prefer, therefore, to consult simply the general convenience of my readers. I think I do so best by considering first the disorders which beset the child in the first month of its existence, during what may be termed its transition from the condition of existence in the womb, to its living, breathing state as an inhabitant of this world; and next the more important ailments to which it is liable during that important time of development which ends with the completion of teething. Afterwards may be studied the diseases of the head, the chest, and the bowels; next constitutional diseases, such as consumption and scrofula; and lastly, the various fevers, as typhoid, or, as it is popularly called, remittent fever, measles, scarlatina, and small-pox; and last of all I will add a few remarks on the mental and moral characteristics of childhood, and their disorders.

CHAPTER IV.

ON THE DISORDERS AND DISEASES OF CHILDREN DURING THE FIRST MONTH AFTER BIRTH.

=Still-birth.=--The infant cries almost as soon as it comes into the world. The cry is the evidence that air has entered its lungs, that the blood has now begun to take a different course from that which it followed before birth, and that the child has entered on a new existence. The child who does not cry, does not breathe; it is said to be still-born; its quietude means death.

After a long or a difficult labour, or after the use of instruments, the child is sometimes still-born in consequence of blood being poured out on its brain, and it is thus killed before birth by apoplexy. This, however, is not usually the case, but the child is generally still-born because some cause or other, generally the protraction of labour, interfered with the due changes of its blood within the womb, and it is born suffocated before its birth, and consequently unable to make the necessary efforts to breathe afterwards.

Drowned people are often resuscitated; the child's case is analogous to theirs; and in both the same measures have to be pursued, namely to try to establish respiration. The degree of the warmth of the child's body, the resistance of its muscles, the red tint or the white colour of its surface, the presence or absence of perceptible beating of its heart, measure the chances of success. Sometimes mere exposure to the cold air produces the necessary effect; at other times breathing is excited by dashing cold water in the child's face, by slapping it, by tickling its nostrils, or by dipping it for a few seconds in a hot bath at 100?or 102? and then swinging it a few times backwards and forwards in the air.

Much time, however, must not be lost over these proceedings, but the child must be laid on its back, the lower part of its body well wrapped up, the chest slightly raised by a folded napkin placed under it. The two arms must then be taken firmly, raised and slowly extended on either side of the head, then brought down again and gently pressed on either side of the chest; and this movement of alternate raising and extending the arms and bringing them back again beside the chest must be repeated regularly some thirty times in the minute, thus imitating the movements of the chest in breathing. These efforts, too, must not be discontinued so long as the surface retains its warmth, and as an occasional heart-beat shows that life is not absolutely extinct; and I believe that in many instances failure is due to want of perseverance rather than to the absolute uselessness of the measure.

=Premature Birth.=--In spite of very extraordinary exceptions, it may be laid down as a rule that children born before the completion of six and a half months of pregnancy do not survive. After that date, each additional week adds greatly to the chances of the child living. There is a mistaken idea, founded on a superstition connected with the number seven, that a seven-months child is more likely to survive than one born at the eighth month. But this notion is as destitute of support in fact as it is opposed to common sense, and the nearer any woman has approached the full term of forty weeks of pregnancy, the greater are the chances of her child being born alive and healthy.

The premature child is by no means necessarily still-born. It breathes, but does so imperfectly, so that air does not enter all the smaller air-cells; and its voice is a whimper rather than a cry. Those changes in the heart and large vessels, which prepare, as pregnancy draws to a close, for the altered course of the blood when the child has to breathe through the lungs, are too little advanced for it to bear well the sudden alteration in its mode of being. The feebly beating heart and the not completely developed lungs seem but imperfectly to maintain the bodily heat. The glands of the stomach and intestines are not yet fit to perform digestion properly, while the muscular power is too feeble for the effort at sucking. Everything is sketched out, but to nothing has the finishing touch been put, and hence the frail machinery too often breaks down, in the endeavour to discharge its functions.

It is surprising, however, with what rapidity Nature in some instances perfects the work which she has been called on prematurely to perform.

It is our business to second Nature's endeavours. First of all, and of most importance, is the duty of providing from without the warmth which the child is unable to generate. When very feeble, it must, even without any previous washing or dressing, be at once wrapped in cotton wool, and then in a hot blanket, and surrounded with hot-water bottles. A tin stomach-warmer filled with hot water is very convenient to place under the blanket on which the child lies. Being too feeble to suck, it must be fed, a few drops at a time, from a small spoon; or still better, if it is able to make any effort at sucking, it may draw its nourishment through a quill. The mother after a premature confinement is almost sure to have no milk with which to nourish her child, at any rate for two or three days. It is, therefore, wise to obtain the help of a woman with a healthy baby. She must be allowed to bring her baby with her, since otherwise her supply of milk would fail, especially if she had no other means of getting rid of it than by the breast-pump or by drawing her breast. Even though she may have her own baby, there are few women who can submit, for more than a very few days, to the artificial emptying their breast without the secretion being either greatly lessened or altogether arrested. This, therefore, must be regarded as a resource available only for a few days, and as the child gains strength every effort must be made to get it to take its mother's breast, if she has any supply, or that of the wet-nurse. If this is found impossible, it will be wisest to give up, at any rate for the present, the attempt to nourish the child from the breast, and to obtain for it asses' milk, which is the best substitute. By no means whatever can more than from a sixth to a fourth part of a pint of milk be obtained either by the breast-pump or by drawing the breast; and since a healthy infant of a few weeks old sucks about two pints of milk in twenty-four hours, it is evident that the supply artificially obtained must after the first few days be utterly inadequate.

I have in cases of extreme weakness in premature children succeeded in preserving them by giving them every two hours for two or three days ten measured drops of raw beef juice, five of brandy, and two teaspoonfuls of breast milk. Medicine has no place in the management of these cases; the question is one entirely of warmth, food, and for a time the judicious use of stimulants.

=Imperfect Expansion of the Lungs.=--Children not premature and perfectly well nourished are yet sometimes feeble, breathe imperfectly, cry weakly, suck difficultly or not at all, and die at the end of a few days. Their lamp of life flickered and went out. Such cases are met with for the most part in conditions similar to those in which children are actually still-born; or now and then they take place when labour has been of unusually short duration, the child hurried into the world too rapidly; while in other instances it is not possible to account for their occurrence.

For a long time the nature of these cases was not understood; but rather more than sixty years ago a German physician discovered that air had entered the lungs but imperfectly; that perhaps a third, perhaps even as much as half, of the lungs had never been dilated, but had remained solid and useless; that in consequence the blood was but half-purified, and vitality therefore but half-sustained. The lungs, however, were found to have undergone no real change; they were not diseased, but if air was blown into them the dark solid patches sunk below the level of the surrounding substance, expanded, grew bright in colour and like a sponge from which the water has been squeezed, and crackled, or crepitated as the technical term is, from the air contained within them.

We breathe in health so without conscious effort that we never realise the fact that, according to the calculation of most competent observers, the mere elasticity of the lungs, independent even of the elasticity of the chest walls, opposes a resistance to each inspiration equal to 150 pounds avoirdupois in the grown man and 120 in the grown woman. The want of breath puts the respiratory muscles into play: the man takes a deep inspiration, and by this unconscious effort, he overcomes the resistance of the chest and the elasticity of the lungs. The new-born infant feels the same want and makes the same effort; but its muscular power is small, and its inspirations are often so feeble as to draw the air in some parts only into the larger tubes, while many of the smaller remain undilated, and much of the lung continues in the state in which it was before birth. The blood being thus but imperfectly purified, all the processes of nutrition go on imperfectly, the vital powers languish, the inspiratory efforts become more and more feeble, while the elasticity of the lung is constantly tending to empty the small cells of air and to oppose its entrance, and next the temperature sinks and the infant dies.

Cases in which this condition of the lungs exists usually present the history of the child from the very first having failed to utter a strong and loud cry like that of other children. Even after breathing has gone on for some time, such children usually appear feeble, and they suck with difficulty, although they often make the effort. An infant thus affected sleeps even more than new-born infants usually do; its voice is very feeble, and rather a whimper than a cry. In the cry of the healthy infant you at once detect two parts--the loud cry, suffering or passionate as the case may be, and the less loud back draught of inspiration. The French have two words for these two sounds--the cri and the reprise. The cri is feeble, the reprise is altogether wanting wherever expansion of the lung has to any considerable extent failed to take place, and you would hail this second sound as the best proof of an improvement in the child's condition.

If you watch the child with a little attention you will see that while the chest moves up and down, it is very little, if at all, dilated by the respiratory movements. The temperature falls, the skin becomes pale, and the lips grow livid, and often slight twitching is observed about the muscles of the face. The difficulty in sucking increases, the cry grows weaker and more whimpering, or even altogether inaudible, while breathing is attended with a slight rattle or a feeble cough, and the convulsive movements return more frequently, and are no longer confined to the face, but affect also the muscles of the extremities. Any sudden movement suffices to bring on these convulsive seizures, but even while perfectly still the child's condition is not uniform, but it will suddenly become convulsed, and during this seizure the respiration will be extremely difficult, and death will seem momentarily impending. In a few minutes, however, all this disturbance ceases, and the extreme weakness of the child, its inability to suck, its feeble cry, and its frequent and imperfect inspirations, are the only abiding indications of the serious disorder from which it suffers. But the other symptoms return again and again, until after the lapse of a few days or a few weeks the infant dies.

I have dwelt at some length on this condition because it is important to know that during the first few weeks of life real inflammation of the lungs or air-tubes is of extremely rare occurrence, and that the symptoms which are not infrequently supposed to depend on it are really due to a portion of the lung more or less extensive never having been called into proper activity. I may add that we shall hereafter have to notice a similar condition of the lung--its collapse after having once been inflated--as occurring sometimes in the course of real inflammation of the organs of respiration in early life, and forming a very serious complication of the original disease.

If the collapse of the lung is not so considerable as to destroy life within the first few hours or days after birth, the babe wastes as well as grows weaker and weaker, and this wasting coupled with the difficult breathing not seldom causes the fear that the child has been born consumptive and that its death is inevitable.

No such gloomy view need be taken. Collapse, or at least non-expansion of the lung to some extent, is by no means unusual: consumptive disease to such an extent in the new-born infant as to interfere with the establishment of breathing is extremely rare. The consumptive babe can suck, it is not so weak as the one whose lungs are imperfectly expanded; it has no convulsive twitchings, nor any of the strange head-symptoms which we notice in the former. It wastes less rapidly, it is feverish instead of having a lower temperature than natural, it seems less ill, and yet its death within a few weeks or months is absolutely certain; while the child whose lungs are not diseased but simply unexpanded may, if that accidental condition is removed, grow up to vigorous manhood.

The treatment of these cases is abundantly simple. The child who breathes imperfectly but ill maintains its heat. It must be kept warm at a temperature never less than 70? it may, like the premature child, need stimulants, and all the precautions already mentioned as to feeding. Twice in the day it should be put for five minutes in a hot bath at 100? rendered even more stimulating by the addition of a little mustard. The back and chest may be rubbed from time to time with a stimulating liniment, and an emetic of ipecacuanha wine may be given twice a day. The act of vomiting not only removes any of the mucus which is apt to accumulate in the larger air tubes, but the powerful inspirations which follow the effort tend to introduce air into the smallest vesicles of the lungs, and to do away with their collapse.

Let these directions be carried out sensibly, patiently, perseveringly, and three times out of four, or oftener still, the mother's ear will before many days be greeted by the loud cry, with its cri and reprise of which I have already spoken, and which assures her that her little one will live.

There are no other affections of the lungs so peculiar to the first month of life as to call for notice here. I shall have a few observations to make about malformations of the heart, and the precautions for which they call in the after-life of children; but they will find their fittest place in the chapter on Affections of the Chest.

=Jaundice of New-born Children.=--A certain yellow tinge of the skin, unattended by any other sign of jaundice, such as the yellowness of the eye and the dark colour of the urine, is by no means to be confounded with real jaundice. It is no real jaundice, but is merely the result of the changes which the blood with which the small vessels of the skin are overcharged at birth is undergoing; the redness fading as bruises fade, through shades of yellow into the genuine flesh colour.

This is no disease, to be treated with the grey powder and the castor oil wherewith the over-busy monthly nurse is always ready. It is a natural process, which the intelligent may watch with interest, with which none but the ignorant will try to interfere.

There is, however, beside this a real jaundice, in which the skin is more deeply stained, the whites of the eyes are yellow, the urine high-coloured, and in which the dark evacuations that carry away the contents of the bowels before birth are succeeded by white motions, from which the bile is absent. This condition is not very usual, save where children have been exposed to cold, or where the air they breathe is unwholesome. Of this no better proof can be given than is afforded by the fact that in the Dublin Lying-in Hospital, where the children are defended with the greatest care both from cold and from a vitiated atmosphere, infantile jaundice is extremely rare, while it attacks three-fourths of the children received into the Foundling Hospital of Paris. Still it does sometimes occur when yet no cause can be assigned for it, and it is noteworthy that it is sometimes met with in successive infants in the same family.

As the respiratory function and that of the skin increase in activity, the jaundice will disappear of its own accord. Great attention must be paid during its continuance to avoid exposure of the child to cold, while no other food than the mother's milk should be given. If the bowels are at all constipated, half a grain of grey powder or a quarter of a grain of calomel may be given, followed by a small dose of castor oil, and the aperient will often seem to hasten the disappearance of the jaundice; but in a large number of cases even this amount of medical interference is not needed.

There is, indeed, a very grave form of jaundice, happily of excessive rarity, due to malformation of the liver, to absence or obstruction of the bile-ducts, and often accompanied with bleeding from the navel. I do but mention it; the intensity and daily deepening of the jaundice, the fruitlessness of all treatment, and the grave illness of the child, even though no bleeding should occur, render it impossible to confound this hopeless condition with the trivial ailment of which I have been speaking.

The next chapter will furnish a fitter place than the present for speaking fully of the Disorders of the Digestive Organs.

I will say now but this: that whatever a mother may do eventually, she avoids grave perils for herself by suckling her infant for the first month; while the health of her child, just launched upon the world, is terribly endangered if fed upon those substitutes for its proper nutriment on which after the lapse of a few weeks it may subsist, may even manage to thrive.

There are some local affections incident to the new-born child concerning which a few words may not be out of place; and first of the

=Ophthalmia of New-born Children.=--It is the cause of the loss of sight of nine-tenths of all persons who, among the poor, are said to have been born blind. In the wealthier classes of society it is comparatively rare, and seldom fails to meet with timely treatment, yet many people scarcely realise its dangerous character, or the extreme rapidity of its course.

It generally begins about the third day after birth with swelling of the lid of one or other eye, though both are soon involved. The eyelids swell rapidly, and if the affection is let alone, they soon put on the appearance of two semi-transparent cushions over the eyes. On separating the lids, which it is often very difficult to do owing to the spasmodic contraction of the muscles, their inner surface is seen to be enormously swollen, bright red, like scarlet velvet, bathed in an abundant yellowish thin secretion, which often squirts out in a jet as the lids are forcibly separated. Great care must be taken not to allow any of this fluid to enter the eye of a bystander, nor to touch his own eye until the fingers have been most carefully washed, since the discharge is highly contagious, and may produce most dangerous inflammation of the eyes of any grown person. The discharge being wiped or washed away, the eye itself may be seen at the bottom of the swelling very red, and its small vessels very blood-shot. By degrees the surface of the eye assumes a deeper red, it loses its brightness and its polish, while the swelling of the lids lessens, and they can be opened with less difficulty; their inner surface at the same time becomes softer, but thick and granular, and next the eyes themselves put on likewise a granular condition which obscures vision. The discharge by this time has become thicker and white, and looks like matter from an abscess. By slow degrees the inflammation may subside, the discharge lessen, the swelling diminish, and the eye in the course of weeks may regain its natural condition. But the danger is--and when proper treatment is not adopted early the danger is very great--lest the mischief should extend beyond the surface of the eye, lest ulceration of the eye should take place, the ulceration reach so deep as to perforate it, and not merely interfere with the sight, but destroy the organ of vision altogether.

In every instance, then, in which the eyelids of a new-born infant swell, or the slightest discharge appears from them, the attention of the doctor must at once be called to the condition. In the meantime, and during whatever treatment he may think it right to follow, the eye must be constantly covered with a piece of folded lint dipped in cold water; and every hour at least the eye must be opened and tepid water squeezed into it abundantly from a sponge held above, but not touching it, so as to completely wash away all the discharge. A weak solution of alum and zinc, as one grain of the latter to three of the former to an ounce of water, may in like manner be dropped from a large camel's-hair brush four times a day into the eye after careful washing. Simple as these measures are they yet suffice, if adopted at the very beginning, and carried on perseveringly, to entirely cure in a few days an ailment which if let alone leads almost always to most lamentable results.

I do not pursue the subject further, for bad cases require all the care of the most skilful oculist for their treatment.

=Scalp Swellings.=--Almost every new-born child has on one or other side of its head a puffy swelling, owing to the pressure to which the head has been subjected in birth, and this swelling disappears at the end of twenty-four or forty-eight hours.

Now and then, however, though indeed very seldom, the swelling does not disappear, but it goes on gradually increasing and becoming more definite in its outlines until at the end of three or four days it may be as big as half a small orange, or sometimes even larger, soft, elastic, painless, under the unchanged scalp, but presenting the peculiarity of having a hard raised margin with a distinct edge, which gives to the finger passed over it the sensation of a bony ridge, beyond which the bone seems deficient. This tumour is due usually to the same cause as that which produces the other temporary puffy swelling of the scalp, only the pressure having been more severe, blood has actually been forced out from the small vessels under the membrane which covers the skull, and hence its gradual increase, its definite outline; and hence, too, the bony ridge which surrounds it, and which is due to nature's effort at cure, in the course of which the raised edge of the membrane covering the skull (the pericranium) becomes converted into bone.

When the nature of these swellings was not understood, they used to be poulticed, and to be opened with a lancet to let out their contents. We know now, however, that we have nothing to do but to let them alone; that by degrees the blood will be absorbed and the tumour will disappear, and as it does so we may trace the gradual transformation of the membrane which covered it into bone, as we feel it crackling like tinsel under the finger. Two, three, or four weeks may be needed for the entire removal of one of these blood-swellings. The doctor will at once recognise its character, and you will then have nothing to do but to wait--often, unhappily, so much harder for the anxious mother than to meddle.

=Ruptured Navel.=--There is a period some time before the birth of a child when the two halves of its body are not united in front, as they become afterwards; and hare-lip or cleft-palate sometimes remains as the result of the arrest of that development which should have closed the fissured lip or united the two halves of the palate.

In a similar way it happens sometimes that though the skin is closed, the muscles of the stomach (or, more properly speaking, of the belly) are not in the close apposition in which they should be, so that the bowels are not supported by the muscles, but protected only by the skin.

More frequently than this, especially in the case of children who are born before the time, the opening through which the navel string passes is large at birth, and fails to close as speedily and completely as it should do afterwards. When everything goes on as it ought, the gradual contraction of the opening helps to bring about the separation of the navel string and its detachment, and the perfect closure of the opening takes place at the same time, between the fifth and the eighth day after birth.

If this does not occur, the bowels are very apt to protrude through the opening, and if allowed to do so for weeks or months, the opening becomes so dilated that its closure is impossible, and the child grows up afflicted permanently with rupture through the navel. This is always an inconvenience, sometimes even a source of serious danger; but if means are taken to prevent the condition becoming worse, nature seldom fails eventually to bring about a cure, and to effect the complete closure of the opening.

If the muscles on either side do not come into apposition, but leave a cleft between them, the infant should constantly wear a broad bandage of fine flannel round the stomach, not applied too tightly, in order to give support. The circular bandages of vulcanised india-rubber with a pad in the centre are nowise to be recommended. The pad is apt to become displaced, and to press anywhere but over the navel, while its edges irritate the infant's delicate skin, and the pressure which it exerts if it is sufficiently tight to retain its place interferes with respiration.

A pad composed of pieces of plaster spread on wash-leather, and of graduated sizes and kept in place by adhesive strapping,[7] answers the purpose of preventing the protrusion at the navel, and of thus facilitating the closure of the ring better than any other device with which I am acquainted. They need, however, to be continued even for two or three years, and though they should have been left off it is wise to resume their use if the child should be attacked by whooping-cough, diarrh[oe]a, or any other ailment likely to occasion violent straining.

FOOTNOTES:

[7] These plasters for ruptured navel in sets of a dozen are to be had of Ewen, 106 Jermyn Street, St. James's, London, and I dare say at many other places besides.

CHAPTER V.

ON THE DISORDERS AND DISEASES OF CHILDREN AFTER THE FIRST MONTH, AND UNTIL TEETHING IS FINISHED.

=Infantile Atrophy.=--In by far the greater number of instances, the wasting of young children is due to their being fed upon food which they cannot digest, or which when digested fails to yield them proper nourishment. I quoted some figures in my introductory remarks, to show from the evidence obtained at Berlin how much larger was the proportion of deaths under the age of one year among hand-fed infants than among those brought up at the breast. Foundling hospitals on the Continent, in which the children are all drawn from the same class, and subjected in all respects to a similar treatment, except that in some they are fed at the breast, in others brought up by hand, show a mortality in the latter case exactly double of that in the former.

It is as idle to ignore these facts, and to adduce in their disproof the case of some child brought up most successfully by hand, as it would be to deny that a battle-field was a place of danger because some people had been present there and had come away unwounded.

But it is always well not merely to accept a fact, but also to know the reason why a thing is so. The reason is twofold: partly because the different substitutes for the mother's milk, taken for the most part from the vegetable kingdom, are less easy of digestion than the milk, and partly because, even were they digested with the same facility, they do not furnish the elements necessary to support life in due proportion.

All food has to answer two distinct purposes: the one to furnish materials for the growth of the body, the other to afford matter for the maintenance of its temperature; and life cannot be supported except on a diet in which the elements of nutrition and those of respiration bear a certain proportion to each other. Now, in milk, the proper food of infants, the elements of the former are to those of the latter about in the proportion of 1 to 2, while in arrowroot, sago, and tapioca they are only as 1 to 26, and in wheaten flour only as 1 to 7. If to this we add the absence in these substances of the oleaginous matters which the milk contributes to supply the body with fat, and the smaller quantity, and to a certain extent the different kind, of the salts which they contain, it becomes apparent that by such a diet the health if not the life of the infant must almost inevitably be sacrificed.

But these substances are not only less nutritious, they are also less easy of digestion than the infant's natural food. We all know how complex is the digestive apparatus of the herbivorous animal, of which the four stomachs of the ruminants are an instance, and how large is the bulk of food in proportion to his size which the elephant requires, compared with that which suffices for the lion or the tiger.

The stomach of the infant is the simple stomach of the carnivorous animal, intended for food which shall not need to stay long in that receptacle, but shall be speedily digested; and it is only as the child grows older, and takes more varied food, that the stomach alters somewhat in form, that it assumes a more rounded shape, resembling somewhat that of the herbivorous animal, and suited to retain the food longer. The young of all creatures live upon their mother for a certain time after birth; but in all the preparation for a different kind of food, and with it for an independent existence, begins much sooner and goes on more rapidly than in man. Young rabbits are always provided with two teeth when born, and the others make their appearance within ten days. In the different ruminants the teeth have either begun to appear before birth, or they show themselves a few days afterwards; and in either case dentition is completed within the first month, and in dogs and cats within the first ten weeks of existence.

In the human subject the process of teething begins late, between the seventh and the ninth month, and goes on slowly: the first grinding teeth are seldom cut before the beginning of the second year, and teething is not finished until after its end. Until teething has begun the child ought to live exclusively on the food which nature provides; for until that time the internal organs have not become fitted to digest other sustenance, and the infant deprived of this too often languishes and dies. To get from other food the necessary amount of nourishment, that food has to be taken in larger quantities, and, from the difficulty in digesting it, needs to remain longer in the stomach than the mother's milk. One of the results of the indigestibility of the food is that the child is often sick, the stomach getting rid of a part of that food which it is unable to turn to any useful purpose; and so far well. But the innutritious substances do not relieve the sense of hunger. The child cries in discomfort, and more is given to it, and by degrees the over-distended stomach becomes permanently dilated, and holds a larger quantity than it was originally meant to contain. The undigested mass passes into a state of fermentation, and the infant's breath becomes sour and offensive, it suffers from wind and acid eructations, and nurses sometimes express surprise that the child does not thrive since it is always hungry. While some of the food is got rid of by vomiting, some passes into the intestines, and there becomes putrid, as the horribly offensive evacuations prove. They come away, large and solid and white, for the secretion of the bile is inadequate to complete that second digestion which should take place in the intestines; or else the irritation which they excite occasions diarrh[oe]a--a green putty-like matter comes away mixed with a profuse watery discharge.

What wonder is it that in such circumstances the body should waste most rapidly; for it is forced from its own tissues to supply those elements essential to the maintenance of life, which its food contains in far too scanty a proportion. Every organ of the body contributes to the general support, and life is thus prolonged, if no kind disease curtail it, until each member has furnished all that it can spare, and then death takes place from starvation, its approach having been slower, but the suffering which preceded it not therefore less, than if all food had been withheld.

Do not suppose that in this description I have been painting too dark a picture, or that children who die thus have been exceptionally weak, and so under the acknowledged difficulties of hand-feeding at length became consumptive. They do not die of consumption, and in a large number of instances their bodies show no trace of consumptive disease, but present appearances characteristic of this condition of starvation, and of this only.

Along the whole track of the stomach and intestines are the signs of irritation and inflammation. The glands of the bowels are enlarged, actual ulceration of the stomach is often met with; while so far-reaching is the influence of this slow starvation, that even the substance of the kidneys and of the brain are often found softened and otherwise altered, though it might not unreasonably have been supposed that these organs lay quite beyond the reach of any disorder of digestion.

No doubt all these grievous results do not always follow; and sometimes children exceptionally strong manage to take and digest enough even of unsuitable food to maintain their health, and may as they grow up, and the changes take place in the system which fit it for a varied diet, even become robust. In the majority of instances, however, hand-fed infants, and those especially who have been brought up chiefly on farinaceous food, are less strong than others, and are more apt to develop any latent tendency to hereditary disease, such as scrofula or consumption, than members of the same family who have been brought up at the breast.

Enough has already been said to satisfy all but those who do not wish to be convinced, how incumbent it is on every mother to try to suckle her child. But though it is most desirable that for the first six months of their existence children should derive their support entirely from their mother, and that until they are a year or at least nine months old their mother's milk should form the chief part of their food, yet many circumstances may occur to render the full adoption of this plan impracticable. In some women the supply of milk, although at first abundant, yet in the course of a few weeks undergoes so considerable a diminution as to become altogether insufficient for the child's support; while in other cases, although its quantity continues undiminished, yet from some defect in its quality it does not furnish the infant with proper nutriment. Cases of the former kind are not unusual in young, tolerably healthy, but not robust women; while instances of the latter are met with chiefly among those who have given birth to several children, whose health is bad, or among the poor, who have been enfeebled by hard living or hard work. The children in the former case thrive well enough for the first six weeks or two months, but then, obtaining the milk in too small a quantity to meet the demands of their rapid growth, they pine and fret, they lose both flesh and strength, and, unless the food given to supply their wants be judiciously selected, their stomach and bowels become disordered, and nutrition, instead of being aided, is more seriously impaired. In the case of the mother whose milk disagrees with the child from some defect in its quality, the signs are in general more pronounced. Either the infant vomits more than that small quantity which a babe who has sucked greedily or overmuch often rejects immediately on leaving the breast, or it is purged, or it seems never satisfied, does not gain flesh, does not thrive, cries much and is not happy. In these cases, too, the mother's supply of milk, though abundant at first, diminishes in a few weeks; she feels exhausted, and suffers from back-ache, or from pain in the breasts each time after the child's sucking; while, further, her general weakness leaves her no alternative but to wean the child.

Knowing the attempt to rear her child entirely at the breast to be vain, the mother may in such cases be tempted to bring it up by hand from the very first. But how short soever the period may be during which the mother may be able to suckle her child, it is very desirable that she should nurse it during that period, and also that her milk should then constitute its only food. For the first four or five days after the infant's birth the milk possesses peculiar qualities, and not merely abounds in fatty and saccharine matter, but presents its casein or curd in a form in which it is specially easy of digestion. These peculiarities indeed become less marked within a week or two; but not only is it of moment that the infant should at any rate make its start in life with every advantage, but the mother who nurses her little one even for a month avoids thereby almost half the risks which follow her confinement. For the indolent, among the wealthy, a numerous class who have but to form a wish in order to have it gratified, a wet-nurse for the baby suggests itself at once to the mother as a ready means of saving herself trouble, and of shirking responsibility. This course, to which love of pleasure and personal vanity tend alike to prompt her, often finds, in spite of all opposing reasons, the approval of the nurse, to whom it saves trouble, and the too ready acquiescence of the doctor in a course which pleases his patient. But many circumstances besides those moral considerations, which ought never to be forgotten before the determination is formed to employ a wet-nurse, may put this expedient out of the question, and it becomes therefore of importance to learn what is the best course for a mother to adopt who is either wholly unable to suckle her child, or who can do so only for a very short time.

It is obvious that the more nearly the substitute approaches to the character of the mother's milk, the greater will be the prospect of the attempt to rear the child upon it proving successful. There is no argument needed to prove that the milk of some animal more closely resembles the mother's milk, and is more likely to prove a useful substitute for it than any kind of farinaceous substance. The milk of all animals, however, differs in many important respects from human milk, and differs too very widely in different animals. Thus, the milk of the cow and that of the ewe contain nearly double the quantity of curd, and that of the goat more than twice the quantity of butter, and it is only in the milk of the ass that the solid constituents are arranged in the same order as in man. On this account, therefore, asses' milk is regarded, and with propriety, as the best substitute for the child's natural food. Unfortunately, however, expense is very frequently a bar to its employment, and compels the use of the less easily digested cows' milk. But though the cost may be a valid objection to the permanent employment of asses' milk, it is yet very desirable when a young infant cannot have the breast, that it should be supplied with asses' milk for the first four or five weeks, until the first dangers of the experiment of bringing it up by hand have been surmounted. The deficiency of asses' milk in butter may be corrected by the addition of about a twentieth part of cream, and its disposition to act on the bowels may be lessened by heating it to boiling point, not over the fire but in a vessel of hot water; and still more effectually by the addition to it of a fourth part of lime-water or of a teaspoonful of the solution of saccharated carbonate of lime to two ounces or four tablespoonfuls of the milk.

When cows' milk is given, it must be borne in mind that it contains nearly twice as much curd, and about an eighth less sugar, than human milk. It is therefore necessary that it should be given in a diluted state and slightly sweetened. The dilution must vary according to the infant's age; at first the milk may be mixed with an equal quantity of water, but as the child grows older the proportion of water may be reduced to one-third. Mere dilution with water, however, leaves the proportion of curd unaltered, and it is precisely the curd which the infant is unable to digest. Instead, therefore, of diluting the milk simply with water, it is often better to add one part of whey to about two parts of milk, which, according to the child's age, may or may not be previously diluted.[8]

Attention must be paid to the temperature of the food when given to the infant, which ought to be as nearly as possible the same as that of the mother's milk, namely from 90?to 95?Fahrenheit, and in all cases in which care is needed a thermometer should be employed in order to insure the food being given at the same temperature. Human milk is alkaline, and even if kept for a considerable time it shows little tendency to become sour. The milk of animals when in perfect health likewise presents an alkaline reaction, and that of cows when at grass forms no exception to this rule. Milk even very slightly acid is certain to disagree with an infant; it is therefore always worth while the moment that a hand-fed infant seems ailing to ascertain this point. If alkaline, the milk will deepen the blue colour of litmus paper, which is to be had of any chemist; if acid, it will discharge the colour and turn it red. It is, perhaps, as well to add that, as the oxygen in the atmosphere tends to redden litmus paper, it should not be left exposed to the air, but should always be kept in a glass-stoppered bottle.

The milk of the cow is very liable to alteration from comparatively slight causes, and particularly from changes in the animal's diet; while even in the most favourable circumstances if the animal is shut up in a city and stall-fed, all the solid constituents of its milk suffer a remarkable diminution; while the secretion further has a great tendency to become acid, or to undergo even more serious deterioration. Mere acidity of the milk can be counteracted for the moment by the addition of lime-water, or by stirring up with it a small quantity of prepared chalk, which may be allowed to subside to the bottom of the vessel; or if it should happen, though indeed that is rarely the case in these circumstances, that the child is constipated, carbonate of magnesia may be substituted for the chalk or lime-water. If these simple proceedings are not sufficient to restore the infant's health, it will be wise to seek at once for another source of milk supply, and to place the suspected milk in the hands of the medical officer of health or of the public analyst, in order that it may be submitted to a thorough chemical and microscopical examination.

The difficulty sometimes found in obtaining an unvaryingly good milk supply, as well as practical convenience in many respects, has led to the extensive employment of various forms of condensed milk. They form undoubtedly the best substitute for fresh cows' milk which we possess, and are a great boon especially to the poor in large towns where the milk supply is often scanty, not always fresh, and sometimes of bad quality. I should certainly prefer condensed milk for an infant to milk from cows living in close dirty stables, such as my experience thirty years ago made me familiar with in some parts of London.

Still all the varieties of condensed milk are far inferior in quality to good fresh milk. They contain less butter, less albumen, that is to say less of the main constituents of all animal solids and fluids, and a greater proportion of what are termed the hydro-carbonates, such for instance as sugar; or, to state the same thing differently, the elements which serve for nutrition are in smaller proportion than in fresh milk to those which minister to respiration. They are not only less nutritious, but the large quantity of sugar which they contain not infrequently disagrees with the child, and causes bowel complaint. I do not know how far the so-called unsweetened condensed milk which has of late come into the market is free from this objection; but I have always preferred the Aylesbury condensed milk, which is manufactured with sugar, to the Swiss condensed milk, into which, as I have been given to understand, honey largely enters.

How much food does an infant of a month old require? what intervals should be allowed between each time of feeding? and how should the food be given? are three questions which call for a moment's notice. The attempt has been made to determine the first point by two very distinguished French physicians, who weighed the infants before and after each time of sucking. Their observations, however, were not sufficiently numerous to be decisive, and their results were very conflicting; the one estimating the quantity at two pounds and a quarter avoirdupois, which would be equivalent to nearly a quart, the other at not quite half as much; but the observations of the latter were made on exceptionally weak and sickly infants. Infants no doubt vary, as do grown people, as to the quantity of food they require. I should estimate from my own experience and observation, apart from accurate data, a pint as the minimum needed by an infant a month old; and while Dr. Frankland's estimate of a pint and a half for an infant of five months seems to me very reasonable, I should doubt its sufficing for a child of nine months unless it were supplemented by other food.

The infant during the first month of life takes food every two hours, and even when asleep should not be allowed to pass more than three hours; and this frequent need of food continues until the age of two, sometimes even until three, months. Afterwards, and until six months old, the child does not need to be fed oftener than every three hours during the twelve waking hours, and every four hours during the sleeping time. Later on, five times in the twenty-four hours, namely thrice by day, once the last thing at night, and once again in the early morning, are best for the child's health as well as for the nurse's comfort.

How is an infant not at the breast to be fed? Certainly not with the cup or spoon; a child so fed has no choice in the matter, but must either swallow or choke, and is fed as they fatten turkeys for the market. The infant, on the other hand, sucks the bottle as it would suck its mother's breast; it rests when fatigued, it stops to play, it leaves off when it has had enough, and many a useful inference may be drawn by the observant nurse or mother who watches the infant sucking, and notices if the child sucks feebly, or leaves off panting from want of breath, or stops in the midst, and cries because its mouth is sore or its gums are tender.

But it is not every bottle which an infant should be fed from, and least of all from those so much in vogue now with the long elastic tube, so handy because they keep the baby quiet, who will lie by the hour together with the end in its mouth, sucking, or making as though it sucked, even when the bottle is empty. These bottles, as well as the tubes connected with them, are most difficult to keep clean; and so serious is this evil, that many French physicians not only denounce their use, in which they are perfectly justified, but prefer, to the use of any bottle at all, the feeding the infant with a spoon; and here I think they are mistaken. The old-fashioned flat bottle, with an opening in the middle, and a short end to which the nipple is attached without any tube, the only one known in the time of our grandmothers, continues still the best, and very good. My friend, Mr. Edmund Owen, in a lecture at which I presided at the Health Exhibition in August last year, pointed out very humorously the differences between the old bottle and the new. An infant to be kept in health must not be always sucking, but must be fed at regular intervals. The careful nurse takes the infant on her knee, feeds it from the old-fashioned feeding-bottle, regulating the flow of the milk according as the infant sucks heartily or slowly, withdraws it for a minute or two, and raises the child into a sitting posture if it seems troubled with flatulence, and then after a pause lets it recommence its meal. This occupies her a quarter of an hour or twenty minutes of well-spent time, while the lazy nurse, or the mother who has never given the matter a thought, just puts the tube in the infant's mouth, and either takes no further trouble or occupies herself with something else. And yet, obvious though this is, how constantly one sees infants taken about in the perambulator with the feeding-bottle wrapped up and laid by its side, because it is said the child always cries when it is not sucking, and the intelligence and the common sense are wanting, as well as the patient love, that would strive to make out which it is of many possible causes that makes the infant cry. One more observation with reference to bottle-feeding may not be out of place. It is this: that no food be left in the bottle after the child has had its meal, but that it should be emptied, washed out with a little warm water and soda, and it and the india-rubber end should be kept in water till again needed. To insure the most perfect cleanliness it is always well to have two bottles in use, and to employ them alternately.

How strictly soever an infant may be kept at the breast, or however exactly the precautions on which I have insisted are observed, sickness, constipation, or diarrh[oe]a may occur, causing much anxiety to the parents, and giving much trouble to the doctor.

It sometimes happens, without its being possible to assign for it any sufficient reason, that the mother's milk disagrees with her infant, or entirely fails to nourish it, so that, much against her will, she is compelled to give up suckling it. In some instances this is due to errors in diet, to the neglect of those rules the observance of which is essential to health, as proper exercise for instance; and then the secretion is usually deficient in quantity as well as defective in its composition. In such cases the child often vomits soon after sucking, it suffers from stomach-ache, its motions are very sour, of the consistence of putty, and either green, or become so soon after being passed, instead of presenting the bright yellow colour and semi-fluid consistence of the evacuations of the healthy infant, and sometimes they are also lumpy from the presence of masses of undigested curd. In addition, also, the child is troubled with griping, which makes it cry; its breath is sour, or actually offensive, and the tongue is much whiter than it should be, though it must be remembered that the tongue of the sucking child always has a very slight coating of whitish mucus, and is neither as red nor as perfectly free from all coating as it becomes in the perfectly healthy child of three or four years old.

In these circumstances, the diminution of stimulants, such as the stout of which young women are sometimes mistakenly urged to take a quantity to which they were previously quite unaccustomed, is often followed by an increase of the quantity as well as an improvement in the quality of the milk. It is true that a nursing mother may often find her strength maintained, and her supply of milk increased, by taking a glass of stout at lunch and another at dinner, instead of, but not in addition to, any other stimulant; but mere stimulants will no more enable a woman to suckle her infant better than she otherwise would do, than they would fit a man to undergo great fatigue for days together, or to go through a walking tour in Switzerland. A tumbler of one-third milk and two-thirds good grit gruel taken three times a day will have greater influence in increasing the quantity of milk than any conceivable amount of stimulant.

There is an entirely opposite condition in which the infant does not thrive at the breast, and this for the most part is met with when the mother has already given birth to and suckled several children. In these instances the secretion is sometimes, though not always, abundant, but the infant does not thrive upon it. The babe does not get on, is always hungry after leaving the breast, and cries as though it wanted more; in addition to which it is often purged, either while sucking or within a few minutes afterwards, though the motions, except in being more frequent and more watery than in health, do not by any means constantly show any other change. The mother's history explains the rest. She is constantly languid, suffers from back-ache, feels exhausted each time after the babe has sucked, probably has neuralgia in her face, or abiding headache. In many instances, too, her monthly periods return, though as a rule they do not appear in healthy women while suckling. All these symptoms show that her system is not equal to the duty she has undertaken, and that therefore, for her sake as well as for that of the infant, she must give up the attempt.

One more case there is in which suckling has to be given up, at any rate in part, and that is when the milk is good in kind, but insufficient in quantity for the child as it grows older. This insufficiency of quantity shows itself at different periods after the infant's birth--at two months, three, or four. The child is not otherwise ill than that it is no longer bright, as it was wont to be, it ceases to gain flesh, it sleeps more than it used to do, though when it wakes it is always eager for the breast, and cries when leaving it, and if the experiment is made of giving it some milk and water immediately on leaving it, it takes that greedily. Mothers are loth to believe this failure of their resources, and in the case of some who have firm and well-formed breasts, there is but little change in their appearance to show that what remains may serve for beauty, not for use. But if while the child is sucking, the nipple is taken suddenly from its mouth, instead of innumerable little jets of milk, spirting out from the openings of the milk-ducts, the nipple will be seen to be barely moistened by its languid flow.

In conditions such as these the question of weaning partially or completely inevitably occurs, and where the mother's weakness is the occasion of the failure to nourish the child, half-measures are of no avail, for so long as she does not entirely give up the attempt to do that to which her health is unequal, her own state will grow worse, that of the child will not improve. When errors of diet or inattention to general rules of health incapacitate the mother from the performance of her duty, there may be hope from the adoption of a wiser course; while when the supply simply fails from its inadequacy, much may be hoped for from a wise combination of hand-feeding with nursing at the breast; the mother perhaps suckling the infant by day, but being undisturbed by demands upon her at night.

Last of all, I must refer to cases in which love has been stronger than reason, as indeed it often is, and in which young people with some pronounced hereditary taint of scrofula or consumption marry and have children. In such cases, if the consumptive taint is on the mother's side, it is, I believe, much wiser, in the inability to obtain a good wet-nurse, to bring up the child by hand rather than at the mother's breast. One word, however, applicable in such circumstances, age and long experience entitle me to add, and it is this. It is essential that, in the absence of that guarantee against the too rapid succession of pregnancies which suckling for a reasonable time presents, there should be self-restraint on both sides, lest the inscription on the young wife's grave should be, as I have too often known it, the same as, in despite of poetry and romance, her biographer assigns as the cause of the death of Petrarch's Laura, that she died worn out crebris partubus, by too many babies.

In all of these cases the rules which I have already given with reference to hand-feeding have to be borne in mind: the preference for asses' milk at first, the careful regulation of the amount of curd in the cows' milk afterwards, increased or diminished by the greater or less proportion of whey mixed with it. Sometimes, however much the quantity of curd or casein may be reduced, the child is yet unable to digest it, for it is firm and not easily acted on by the juices of the stomach. It is then best to omit it altogether, and to supply the necessary albumen by white of egg. A very good food in these circumstances is made of--

White of one raw egg, Quarter of an ounce of sugar of milk, Three teaspoonfuls of cream, Half a pint of whey.

In the course of a few weeks, or when the child seems to need stronger nourishment, one part of veal-tea, made with a pound of veal to a pint of water, may be added to one part of whey, with the white of egg and sugar of milk as before, and one part of white decoction, as it was called some two centuries ago in England. It is composed of--

Half an ounce of hartshorn shavings, Inside of one French roll, Three pints of water--boiled to two, strained and sweetened.

This forms an extremely useful way of introducing farinaceous food into the infant's diet, and preparing the way for a larger amount of it which by degrees becomes necessary. Of these, one of the most generally useful is Liebig's or Savory and Moore's food for infants, which has the advantage of not constipating as so many other farinaceous foods do. Chapman's Entire Wheat Flour is an extremely good food; and wheat, as you will remember, excels other farinaceous substances in its nutritive properties, but it is not so easy of digestion as Liebig. There is, however, scarcely any kind of farinaceous food, among which Nestl?s must not be forgotten, which may not answer for an infant; provided always that at first it is not given oftener than twice a day, that it is not made too thick, nor given in larger proportion than one-third of the farinaceous food to two-thirds of the whey, milk, or whatever it is mixed with; and besides, whatever the food may be, it should be prepared each time afresh.

This is not the place for going into all details on the subject of feeding infants, or to explain how if wisely managed the child weans itself by degrees from the bottle or the breast--the best way, be it said, of weaning--or how by degrees it comes to its daily midday meal of beef-tea and bread, and then, when the first grinding teeth have been cut, to a small meat meal daily, finely minced or scraped, and so little by little adopts the modes of living of its elders.

But, last of all, there are instances, though not so many as the public imagine, in which the infant, in spite of most judicious management, fails to thrive, and suffers from various disorders of its digestion.

The most unmanageable and the least hopeful of these cases are those in which the infant is the subject of consumptive disease. It is very rare for its symptoms, even in cases of the most marked tendency to consumption on the part of the parents, to show themselves before the age of three months, and I think I may add, that apart from such tendency consumption never appears in infancy or early childhood, except when it follows on some acute illness, such as inflammation of the lungs, or on typhoid, or, as it is commonly called, remittent fever.

Consumption of the bowels, as it is popularly termed, may be said never to occur in early infancy apart from consumptive disease of the lungs, and is then always accompanied by an increase towards evening of the temperature from its natural standard of 98.5?to 100? Hence the absence of cough and the persistence of a natural temperature may be taken as almost conclusive evidence that there is no consumptive disease of the bowels. Consumptive disease in infancy is invariably attended with glandular enlargement. The glands of the bowels when irritated always communicate their irritation to the glands in the groin and the bend of the thigh, which are felt hard and enlarged, like little peas, under the finger. But further, if there is real disease of the glands of the bowels, other tiny enlarged glands will be felt, like shot, under the skin of the belly, from which in the general progress of emaciation the layer of fat always present in the healthy baby will already have been removed. Besides this, too, the veins running beneath the skin there, invisible in the healthy infant, will be seen meandering like blue lines, and telling the story that more blood than usual flows through them, because the diseased glands inside interfere with its ready passage through its proper channels.

Two cautions, however, have to be borne in mind with reference to both of these indications of disease. The first is, that the glands in the groin may be enlarged from mere irritation, independent of actual disease communicated to them from the glands inside. If, however, you find the glands at the corner of the lower jaw and those on either side of the neck enlarged too, you are then driven to the conclusion that the glands in the groin are enlarged not from mere local irritation, but from general disease, and that consumption is its cause.

Again, the superficial veins of the belly may be enlarged from any cause which interferes with the proper circulation through the vessels inside. Hence they are often enlarged in grown people in dropsy, and hence too in infants and young children from flatulent distension of the bowels. But in this case the other signs of consumption are wanting; the emaciation, the cough, the increase of evening temperature, and the enlargement of the glands, are all absent.

Sometimes we meet with instances where the child does not digest its food, does not thrive, does not gain flesh, never passes healthy evacuations, at length wastes, loses strength, and dies, without having had any of the signs which I have pointed out as indicative of consumptive disease, and in fact without having suffered from it. Now, these cases are connected with imperfect performance of the function of the liver, and sometimes with an imperfection of its structure. Before birth the functions of the liver are not called into action in the same way nor to the same degree as afterwards, and its structure differs in this respect that it contains a larger amount of fat and a smaller proportion of bile-secreting cells than afterwards. It sometimes happens from causes which we do not understand that the liver structure not only does not undergo that higher development which should take place, but that the fat cells increase at the expense of the bile cells. In these circumstances the food is ill-digested and the health is much impaired, and at last wasting takes place to as great a degree as in the case of consumption, only there are no cough, no glandular enlargement, no big superficial veins, no increased temperature, while on a careful examination the doctor will seldom fail to find the rounded edge of the enlarged liver coming lower down than natural. In these cases too there is a disposition to convulsive affections, and to that peculiar form of convulsion called spasmodic croup, concerning which I shall have something to say later on.

In its less serious form this is both a more frequent and a less grave condition than consumption, and its existence explains to a great degree those cases in which young children have failed to be nourished by the milk food which commonly suits their tender age, but have improved on beef-tea, raw meat or its juice, and food entirely destitute of saccharine matter.

In cases where there is reason to apprehend consumptive disease, the skill and resources of the doctor will often be heavily taxed to meet each difficulty as it arises. A good wet-nurse, or, in default of her, asses' milk, with the addition of cream to supply the butter in which the asses' milk is deficient, a couple of teaspoonfuls of raw meat juice in the course of every twenty-four hours, much care in the introduction of farinaceous substances into the diet, and cod-liver oil twice a day, beginning with ten drops and gradually increasing the dose to a teaspoonful, are all that the mother herself can do. When the cod-liver oil is not borne by the stomach, or when--which, however, is not often the case--the child refuses to take it, glycerine may be substituted for it, though it must be owned that it is a very poor and inefficient substitute. The inunction of cod-liver oil is in any case not to be had recourse to; it makes the child unpleasant to itself and loathsome to others, while the power of the skin to absorb oily matters is far too limited to be worth taking into account.

Vomiting, though by no means a prominent symptom of either of the two very grave conditions of which I have been speaking just now, is yet a very common attendant on all disorders of digestion in early life. It is indeed much more frequent in the infant than in the adult, and the greater irritability of the stomach continues even after the first few months of existence are past, and does not completely cease during the early years of childhood. In every case of vomiting in childhood, therefore, the first question to set at rest is whether it depends on disorder of the digestive system, or whether it heralds the onset of one of the eruptive fevers, or of inflammation of the chest, or of affection of the brain; and in determining this all the directions given when I was speaking of the general symptoms of disease are to be carefully studied. Vomiting often accompanies infantile diarrh[oe]a, even when the food taken cannot be regarded as its occasion; and now and then the stomach, with no obvious exciting cause, suddenly becomes too irritable to retain any food, and this indeed may be the case even though attended by few or no other indications of intestinal disorder. The child in such cases seems still anxious for the breast; but so great is the irritability of the stomach that the milk is either thrown up unchanged immediately after it has been swallowed, or it is retained only for a few minutes, and is then rejected in a curdled state; while each application of the child to the breast is followed by the same result. It will generally be found, when this accident takes place in the previously healthy child of a healthy mother, that it has been occasioned by some act of indiscretion on the part of its mother or nurse. She perhaps has been absent from her nursling longer than usual, and returning tired from a long walk or from some fatiguing occupation, has at once offered it the breast, and allowed it to suck abundantly; or the infant has been roused from sleep before its customary hour, or it has been over-excited or over-wearied at play, or in hot weather has been carried about in the sun without proper protection from its rays.

The infant in whom from any of these causes vomiting has come on, must at once be taken from the breast, and for a couple of hours neither food nor medicine should be given to it. It may then be offered a teaspoonful of cold water; and should the stomach retain this, one or two spoonfuls may be given in the course of the next half-hour. If this is not rejected, a little isinglass may be dissolved in the water, which must still be given by a teaspoonful at a time, frequently repeated; or cold barley-water may be given in the same manner. In eight or ten hours, if no return of vomiting takes place, the experiment may be tried of giving the child its mother's milk, or cows' milk diluted with water, in small quantities from a teaspoon. If the food thus given does not occasion sickness, the infant may in from twelve to twenty-four hours be restored to the breast: with the precaution, however, of allowing it to suck only very small quantities at a time, lest, the stomach being overloaded, the vomiting should again be produced.

In many instances when the sickness has arisen from some accidental cause, such as those above referred to, the adoption of these precautions will suffice to restore the child's health. If, however, other signs of disorder of the stomach or bowels have preceded the sickness, or are associated with it, medicine cannot be wholly dispensed with, and the advice of the doctor must be sought for. Very likely in addition to directing the rules above laid down to be attended to, he may lay a tiny dose of calomel, as a quarter, half or a whole grain on the tongue, which often has a wonderful influence in arresting sickness; while he may further put a small poultice not much bigger than a crown piece, made half of mustard, half of flour, on the pit of the stomach for a few minutes, and may give the child a little saline, with a grain or two of carbonate of soda, and perhaps a drop of prussic acid. These, however, are not remedies to be employed by the mother, but must be prescribed, and their effect watched by the medical attendant.

Sickness, indeed, is not always a solitary symptom unattended by other evidences of disordered digestion, but is sometimes associated with signs of its general impairment, and this may be so serious as to lead to great loss of flesh, and even to end in endangering life. In many instances, however, the child does not lose much flesh though it digests ill, and its symptoms would be troublesome rather than alarming, if it were not that they are often the signs of an unhealthy constitution, out of which in the course of a few months consumption is not infrequently developed. Long-continued indigestion in the infant always warrants anxiety on the part of the parent.

In some of these cases there is complete loss of appetite, the infant caring neither for the breast nor for any other food. It loses the look of health and grows pale and languid, though it may not have any special disorder either of the stomach or of the bowels. It sucks but seldom and is soon satisfied, and even of the small quantity taken, a portion is often regurgitated almost immediately. This state of things is sometimes brought on by a mother's over-anxious care, who, fearful of her infant taking cold, keeps it in a room too hot or too imperfectly ventilated. It follows, also, in delicate infants on attacks of catarrh or of diarrh[oe]a, but it is then for the most part a passing evil which time will cure. In the majority of cases, however, the loss of appetite is associated with evidence of the stomach's inability to digest even the small quantity of food taken, and the bowels are irregular in their action, as well as unhealthy in their secretion. Loss of appetite, too, though a frequent is by no means a constant attendant on infantile indigestion, but is replaced sometimes by an unnatural craving, in which the child never seems so comfortable as when sucking. It sucks much, but the milk evidently does not sit well upon the stomach; for soon after sucking, the child begins to cry and appears to be in much pain until it has vomited. The rejection of the milk is followed by immediate relief; but at the same time by the desire for more food, and the child often can be pacified only by allowing it to suck again. In other cases vomiting is of much less frequent occurrence, and there is neither craving desire for food, nor much pain after sucking; but the infant is distressed by frequent acid or offensive eructations; its breath has a sour or nauseous smell, and its evacuations have a most f[oe]tid odour. The condition of the bowels that exists in connection with these different forms of indigestion is variable. In cases of simple loss of appetite, the debility of the stomach is participated in by the intestines, and constipation is of frequent occurrence, though the evacuations do not always appear unhealthy. In other instances in which the desire for food still continues, the bowels may act with due regularity, but the motions may have a very unnatural appearance. If the child is brought up entirely at the breast, the motions are usually liquid, of a very pale yellow colour, often extremely offensive, and contain shreds of curdled milk, which not having been digested within the stomach, pass unchanged through the whole track of the bowels. In many instances, however, the infant having been observed not to thrive at the breast, arrowroot or other farinaceous food is given to it, which the stomach is wholly unable to digest, and which gives to the motions the appearance of putty or pipe-clay, besmeared more or less abundantly with slime or mucus. The evacuations are often parti-coloured, and sometimes one or two unhealthy motions are followed by others which appear perfectly natural; while attacks of diarrh[oe]a often come on, and the matters discharged are then watery, of a dark dirty green colour, and exceedingly offensive.

Children, like grown persons suffering from indigestion, often continue, as I have already said, to keep up their flesh much better than could be expected, and in many cases grow up to be strong and healthy. Still the condition is one that not merely entails much suffering on the infant, but by its continuance seriously impairs the health, and tends to develop the seeds of any constitutional predisposition to consumptive disease.

In these cases there are many respects in which the mother can most efficiently second the doctor. All causes unfavourable to health must be examined into, and as far as possible removed. It must be seen that the nursery is well ventilated, and that its temperature is not too high; while it will often be found that no remedy is half so efficacious as change of air. Next, it must not be forgotten that the regurgitation of the food is due in great measure to the weakness and consequent irritability of the stomach, and care must therefore be taken not to overload it. If these two points are attended to, benefit may then be looked for from the employment of tonics, and as the general health improves the constipated condition of the bowels, so usual in these cases, will by degrees disappear; while if aperients are needed those simple remedies only should be employed of which I spoke in the first part of this book, and the use of mercurials is not to be resorted to without distinct medical order.

The above mode of treatment is appropriate to cases of what may be termed the indigestion of debility, but a different plan must be adopted in those instances in which it depends on some other cause. The rule, indeed, which limits the quantity of food to be given at one time is no less applicable here, for the rejection of some of the milk may be the result of nothing more than of an effort which nature makes to reduce the work that the stomach has to do within the powers of that organ. But when, notwithstanding that due attention is paid to this important point, uneasiness is always produced by taking food, and is not relieved till after the lapse of some twenty minutes, when vomiting takes place, or when the infant suffers much from flatulence and from frequent acid or nauseous eructations, it is clear that the symptoms are due to something more than the mere feebleness of the system.

It is not, however, the mere fact that the child vomits its food, or of the milk so vomited being rejected in a coagulated state, which proves that the stomach is disordered, but it is the fact of firmly coagulated milk being rejected with much pain, and after the lapse of a considerable interval from the time of its being taken, which warrants this conclusion. The coagulation of the curd is the first change which the milk of any animal undergoes when introduced into the stomach. The coagulum of human milk is soft and flocculent, and not so thoroughly separated from the other elements of the fluid, as the firm hard coagulum or curd of cow's milk becomes from the whey in which it floats. In a state of health the abundantly secreted gastric juice speedily redissolves the chief part of the curd in the stomach, while when it has passed into the intestine the alkaline bile which there becomes mixed with it, completes its solution, and converts the whole into a fluid which closely resembles one of the chief elements of the blood, is consequently very easily taken up by the minute vessels whose office it is to do so, and thus supplies with nourishment the whole body.

Milk tends, however, to undergo changes spontaneously, which produce its coagulation, and the occurrence of these changes is greatly favoured by a moderately high temperature, such as that which exists in the stomach. But the alterations of the fluid that accompany this spontaneous coagulation are very different from those which are brought about by the vital processes of digestion. An acid becomes formed within it, and the acid thus produced has none of the solvent power of gastric juice, but by its presence impedes rather than favours digestion. Every nurse is aware that a very slight acidity of the milk will suffice to give an infant vomiting, stomach ache, and diarrh[oe]a, and the result must be much the same whether fermentation had begun in the milk before it was swallowed, or whether it commences afterwards, in consequence of the disordered condition of the stomach, and the absence of a healthy secretion of gastric juice.

The nature of the food is the first point that requires attention in the management of these cases of infantile dyspepsia. If the child had been fed on cow's milk the symptoms may be due to the gastric juice not having been able to dissolve the curd, which you will remember is much firmer than that of human milk as well as twice as abundant. In this case the substitution of asses' milk, the employing whey either entirely or in part instead of milk, and the adding white of egg in order to present the elements of the curd in a more easily digestible form, may all be tried with advantage. Sometimes children refuse whey; and then a mixture of cream and veal broth, more or less diluted either with water or with the white decoction, may be given instead. The addition of soda, potash, chalk or lime water to milk before it is given is also of service, since it not only prevents the occurrence of fermentation, but also renders the curd of cow's milk more easily soluble.

The indiscriminate and over-free employment of these alkalies, however, as nursery remedies is by all means to be avoided, for the symptoms of indigestion for which a grown person if suffering would seek the advice of a skilful doctor require his help no less when the patient is a child. When acids will be of service in promoting the secretion of the gastric juice, when pepsine will be likely to be of use, when stimulants such as a little brandy, when aromatics to get rid of flatulence, opiates to relieve pain or check diarrh[oe]a, or when an occasional mercurial, or some other remedy may be of use by stimulating the liver to increased action, are questions which I would not advise any mother to try to answer for herself. Much care and pains and knowledge and experience are often required by the doctor to enable him to answer them correctly.

I must not leave the consideration of the ailments of the digestive organs in early infancy without some notice of that affection of the mouth popularly known as thrush to which an exaggerated importance was once attached as the supposed cause of those symptoms of disordered health, of which it is in reality only the accompaniment. Still it is a sign of such grave disorder that it needs a careful study.

THRUSH.--If you examine the mouth of a young infant, in whom the attempt at hand-feeding is not turning out well, you will often observe its lining to be beset with numerous small white spots, that look like little bits of curd lying upon its surface, but which on a more attentive examination are found to be so firmly adherent to it as not to be removed without some difficulty, when they leave the surface beneath it a deep red colour, and now and then bleeding slightly. These specks appear upon the inner surface of the lips, especially near the angles of the mouth, on the inside of the cheeks, and upon the tongue, where they are more numerous at the tip and edges than towards the centre. They are likewise seen upon the gums, though less frequently and in smaller numbers. When they first appear they are usually of a circular form, scarcely larger than a small pin's head; but after having existed for a day or two, some of the spots become three or four times as large, while at the same time they in general lose something of their circular form. By degrees the small white crusts fall off of their own accord, leaving the surface where they were seated redder than before; a colour which gradually subsides, as with the infant's improved health the mouth returns to its natural condition. If the improvement is tardy the white specks may be reproduced and again detached several times before the mouth resumes its healthy aspect. In the worst cases the specks coalesce, and coat the mouth as though lined with a membrane which is usually of a yellowish-white tint instead of having the dead white colour of the separate spots. Even here, however, though the surface is very red, it scarcely bleeds if the deposit is removed from it gently and with care.

The popular notion that when the deposit of thrush appears not only in the mouth, but also at the edge of the bowel, it has passed through the child is altogether erroneous. The lining membrane of the bowel indeed is red, inflamed, and presents those conditions to which I have already referred when speaking of the atrophy of hand-fed children, but the actual deposit of thrush can take place only where there exists an appropriate structure for its formation, and that is to be found, not in the bowels, but only at the inlets and outlets of the digestive canal. The actual deposit at the outlet of the bowel is indeed exceptional, though the edges are often red and sore from the irritation produced by the acrid motions, and this irritation sometimes extends to the skin over the lower part of the baby's person, which becomes rough, and covered with a blush of redness.

Thrush in the child is of far less serious import than in the grown person. In the latter it indicates the existence of some very serious, almost hopeless disease, and hence it is that we meet with it in the last stages of dysentery, cancer, and consumption. In the child a slight attack of thrush may occur from causes which are by no means serious, and may disappear under the use of simple means, such as I have already described when speaking of the troubles of digestion in early infancy.

While in any case it must rest with the doctor to regulate as he best knows how the constitutional treatment of the condition on which the thrush depends, it must be for the mother to see that appropriate local measures are adopted. One point of considerable moment, and to which less care than it deserves is usually paid, is the removing from the mouth, each time after the infant has been fed, of all remains of the milk or other food. For this purpose whenever the least sign of thrush appears, the mouth should be carefully wiped out with a piece of soft rag dipped in a little warm water every time after food has been given. Supposing the attack to be but slight this precaution will of itself suffice in many instances to remove all traces of the affection in two or three days. If, however, there is much redness of the mouth, or if the specks of thrush are numerous, some medicated application is desirable.

The once popular honey and borax is not the best application, and this for a reason which I will at once explain. The secretion of the mouth in infants is acid, disease increases this acidity; and it has been found that this acid state is not merely favourable to the increase of thrush, but also to the development between the specks of thrush of a sort of membrane formed by a peculiar microscopic growth, of whose existence, just as of that of the phylloxera which destroys the vine, or the muscardine which kills the silkworm, we were ignorant till brought to light by recent scientific research.

You will therefore at once see why saccharine substances, apt as they are to pass into a state of fermentation, are not suitable, and why it is better to employ a solution of--

Borax, twenty grains Glycerine, one teaspoonful Water, an ounce.

Now and then the use once or twice a day in addition of a very weak solution of caustic, as two grains of lunar caustic to an ounce of water, in bad cases is necessary; but of this it must be left to the doctor to decide.

TEETHING.--The transition is a very natural one by which we pass from the study of the dangers and difficulties which attend the feeding and rearing of young infants, to those which accompany teething.

The time of teething is looked forward to by most mothers with undisguised apprehension, nurses attribute to it the most varied forms of constitutional disturbance, and doctors constantly hold forth to anxious parents the expectation that their child will have better health when it has cut all its teeth. The time of teething, too, is in reality one of more than ordinary peril,[9] though why it should be so is not always rightly understood. It is a time of most active development, a time of transition from one mode of being to another, in respect of all those important functions by whose due performance the body is nourished and built up.

The error which has been committed with reference to this matter, consists not in overrating the hazard of the time, when changes so important are being accomplished, but in regarding only one of the manifestations--though that indeed is the most striking one of the many important ends which nature is then labouring to bring about. A child in perfect health usually cuts its teeth at a certain time and in a certain order, just as a girl at a certain age begins to show signs of approaching womanhood; and at length attains it with but slight inconvenience or discomfort. The two processes, however, have this in common, that during both, constitutional disturbance is more common, and serious diseases are more frequent than at other times, and the cause in both lies far deeper than the outward manifestation.

The great changes which nature is constantly bringing about around us and within us are the result of laws operating silently but unceasingly; and hence it is that in her works we see little of the failure which often disappoints human endeavours, or of the dangers which often attend on their accomplishment. Thus when her object is to render the child no longer dependent on the mother for its food, she begins to prepare for this long beforehand. The first indication of it is furnished by the greatly increased activity of the salivary glands, which during the first few months of existence have scarcely begun to perform their function, a fact which accounts for the tendency to dryness of the tongue of the young infant under the influence of very trivial ailments. About the fourth or fifth month, this condition undergoes a marked alteration; the mouth is now found continually full of saliva, and the child is constantly drivelling; but no other indication appears of the approach of the teeth to the surface, except that the ridge of the gums sometimes becomes broader than it was before. No further change may take place for many weeks; and it is generally near the end of the seventh month before the first teeth make their appearance. The middle cutting teeth of the lower jaw are in most instances the first to pierce the gum; next the middle cutting teeth of the upper jaw; then usually the side cutting teeth of the lower jaw, and lastly, the corresponding ones of the upper. This, however, is not quite invariable, for sometimes all the cutting teeth in one jaw precede in their appearance any of those in the other. The first four grinding teeth next succeed, and often without any very definite order as to whether those of the upper or of the lower jaw are first visible, though in the majority of instances the lower are the first to appear. The four eye teeth follow, and lastly, the remaining four grinding teeth, which complete the set of first, or as they are often called, milk teeth.

We must not, however, picture to ourselves this process as going on uninterruptedly until completed--a mistake into which parents often fall, whose anxiety respecting their children is excited by observing that after several teeth have appeared in rapid succession, the process appears to come to a standstill. Nature has so ordered it that teething which begins at the seventh or eighth month, shall not be completed until the twenty-fourth or thirtieth; and has doubtless done so in some measure with the view of diminishing the risk of constitutional disturbance that might be incurred if the evolution of the teeth went on without a pause. As a rule the two lower central incisors or cutting teeth make their appearance in the course of a week; six weeks or two months often intervene before the central upper incisors pierce the gum, but they are in general quickly followed by the lateral incisors. A pause of three or four months most frequently occurs before we see the first grinding teeth, another of equal length previous to the appearance of the eye teeth, and then another still longer before the last grinding teeth are cut.

Though a perfectly natural process, teething is almost always attended with some degree of suffering. This, however, is not always the case, for sometimes we discover that an infant has cut a tooth, who yet had shown no signs of discomfort, nor any indication that teething was commencing, with the exception of an increased flow of saliva. More frequently indeed, the mouth becomes hot, and the gums look tumid, tense, and shining, while the exact position of each tooth is marked, for some time before its appearance, by the prominence of the gum; or the eruption of the teeth is preceded by much redness, and great heat of the mouth with profuse flow of saliva, and even with little painful ulcers of the edge of the tongue, or of the inner surface of either lip. With either of these conditions the child is feverish, fretful, and cries from time to time with pain, while at the same time the bowels often are relaxed, or the child coughs and wheezes as if it had caught cold.

Symptoms such as these make up what nurses mean when they say that the child is suffering from its teeth, and this opinion is constantly followed by a request to the doctor to lance the baby's gums. Now this little operation when really called for often gives great relief, both to the local discomfort, and also to the general ailment from which the infant suffers, but it is often done when there is no occasion for it, and when consequently it causes needless pain, and does no good.

There are four different conditions in which it may be right to have the child's gums lanced:

First. When a tooth is very near the surface, and by cutting through the thin gum the child may be spared some needless suffering.

Second. When the gums are very red and hot and swollen; only in this case the gum is scratched or cut, to bleed it, not with the idea of letting out the imprisoned tooth.

Third. When the child has for some week or two been feverish and suffering; while, though the gum is tense and swollen, the tooth does not seem to advance.

Fourth. As an experiment, when during the progress of teething a child is suddenly seized with convulsions for which there is no obvious cause. The irritation of the teeth may have to do with their occurrence; and the chance of relieving it by so simple a means is not to be thrown away.

If the process of teething is going on quite naturally, no interference, medical or other, is either necessary or proper. The special liability of children to illness at this time must indeed be borne in mind, and care must be taken not to make any alteration in the infant's food while it is actually cutting its teeth, but rather to choose the opportunity of some one of those pauses to which reference has been made, as occurring between the dates of appearance of the successive teeth, for making any such change. If the child is feverish, a little soda or seltzer water sweetened and given after the effervescence has subsided will be taken eagerly, and avoid the risk of putting the child too often to the breast, or giving it food too frequently. It seeks the one or the other because it is thirsty, and craves for moisture to relieve its hot mouth; not because it is hungry and needs nourishment. If the child has been weaned, still greater care will be required, for it will often be found that it is no longer able to digest its ordinary food, which either is at once rejected by the stomach, or else passes through the intestines undigested. Very thin arrowroot made with water, with the addition of one third of milk, will suit in many cases, or equal parts of milk and water with isinglass, or equal parts of milk and the white decoction. The bowels of course must be kept open with very simple and mild aperients, but the bowels are in general more inclined to diarrh[oe]a than to constipation, and the diarrh[oe]a of teething children is often troublesome and requires good medical advice.

The ulcerated state of the mouth is usually connected with special disorder of the digestive organs, and that condition of acidity for which I have already recommended soda, magnesia, and similar remedies, while locally the mouth needs just that local care which is applicable in cases of thrush. Now and then, severe inflammation of the gums occurs, in which they become extremely swollen; and ulceration takes place of the gum just above where the tooth should come through, and even around some of those which have already appeared. These are cases in which lancing the gums would do nothing but mischief. They require the local care already insisted on, a mild plan of diet, and treatment to reduce any feverishness; and above all one medicine, the chlorate of potass, which in doses of four grains every four hours for a child a year old, is almost a specific.

AFFECTIONS OF THE SKIN.--There are a few affections of the skin to which children in early infancy are especially liable, concerning which a few words must be said.

The Latin word intertrigo is used for that chafing of the skin of the lower part of the body of an infant which is by no means unusual, and is often very distressing. It is almost invariably due to want of care. Either wetted napkins are dried, and put on again without previous rinsing in water, or they have been washed in water containing soda, and not passed through pure water afterwards, or attention is not paid to change the infant's napkin immediately that it requires; or a fresh napkin is put on without previous careful ablution of the child; or lastly it occurs almost unavoidably in cases of diarrh[oe]a from the extension of irritation beginning at the edge of the bowel.

Care is usually all that is needed to remove, as it is to prevent this condition. The precautions which I have referred to with regard to cleanliness must be carefully observed, and moreover, each time even after passing water, the child should be carefully washed with thin gruel, or barley water, then dusted abundantly with starch powder, while the napkin must be thickly greased with zinc ointment. After the first six or seven months of life the napkin can be almost always dispensed with, if the child has been brought up in good habits, and in all cases of chafing, it is much the better way to put no napkin on the child when in bed, but to lay under it a folded towel, which can be removed, and a clean one substituted for it as soon as it becomes soiled.

There is a very obstinate form of chafing, with great redness of the skin, and disposition to crack about the edge of the bowel which depends on constitutional causes, and calls at once for the interference of the doctor.

Besides this purely local ailment, there is another skin affection which is seen over the body generally, and is known popularly by the name of red gum, or in Latin strophulus. I mention the Latin name because I have known persons sometimes, misled by the similarity of sound, fancy that it had some connection with scrofula. It is met with less commonly now than formerly, when people were accustomed to keep infants unduly wrapped up, and to be less careful than most are now-a-days about washing and bathing. It depends on over-irritation of the sweat glands of the delicate skin of the infant, the result of which shows itself in the eruption on the body and face of a number of small dry pimples sometimes surrounded by a little redness, itching considerably, and when their top has been rubbed off by scratching having a little speck of dried blood at their summit.

A rash like this, a sort of nettle rash, more blotchy and causing little lumps on the skin, which in a day or two come and go, sometimes appears in the intervals between the pimples, sometimes takes their place, and causes, as they do, much irritation. This nettle rash is usually dependent on some error of diet, on some acidity of the stomach, and, on their being corrected soon passes away, leaving the pimples as they were before, but sometimes being reproduced if the pimples cause excessive irritation of the tender skin.

The matter of chief importance for a mother to know, is that these rashes have no serious signification. Their treatment is very simple. It consists in dressing the child very lightly, in bathing it very frequently with tepid water, avoiding as far as may be the use of soap, and in sponging it often to relieve the irritation with some simple alkaline lotion; such for instance as one recommended by the late Dr. Tilbury Fox, and which is composed of twenty grains of carbonate of soda, two teaspoonfuls of glycerine, and six ounces of rose water. Of course if the stomach is out of order that must be attended to, but a little fluid magnesia, once or twice a day, is all that is usually needed in the way of medicine.

One other affection of the skin, very common, very distressing, very tedious, of which there are many varieties, generally known by the technical name of eczema, from a compound Greek word which signifies to flow, needs that I should say something about it. It is not limited in its occurrence to infancy, nor does it of necessity cease when childhood is over, but continues to recur even in grown persons, and shows itself still from time to time even in the aged.

For the most part, however, it makes its appearance between the fifth and twelfth month; sometimes seeming to be induced by the change of food when the child is weaned, and that even though the weaning may have been wisely managed; at other times showing itself when the irritation of teething begins, and in every instance being aggravated by the approach of each tooth to the surface, and abating in the intervals.

It does not occur in all children with equal frequency or severity, and though there is no doubt but that it is often hereditary, and this especially in families some members of which have suffered from gout, yet it is by no means unusual for two or three of the children of the same parents to be affected by it severely, while no trace of it appears in the others.

It shows itself in general first on the cheeks and sides of the face, where the skin becomes red and rough, and slightly puffy. On looking very closely--more closely indeed than most persons are wont to do--this appearance will be seen to be produced by innumerable small pimples, smaller than pins' heads, and which itch violently. Now and then, even in the course of a few hours, these pimples disappear, leaving the skin rough, and peeling off in branny scales, while the surface beneath is red and irritable, a condition which also in a few days may subside. This, however, is less frequent than the opposite course of the affection, in which a drop of fluid forms at the top of each tiny pimple, and escaping forms a yellowish, thin, transparent, watery, irritating discharge, which reddens still more the raw and weeping surface of the skin. The fluid when abundant dries at length into yellowish flakes or crusts, which sometimes assume a brownish colour if the surface is made to bleed by irritating or scratching. If the crusts are not removed, the fluid which still continues to be poured out beneath them soon changes into matter or pus as it is called, and this, shut up beneath the hard crust above, increases the irritation, and thickens the deposit. After a time the inflammation lessens of its own accord, the secretion diminishes, the crusts dry up, and at length fall off, leaving the skin red, slightly swollen, and its surface scaling off in flakes, which gradually cease to form, and the skin by degrees becomes quite sound again, and so remains, until perhaps the irritation caused by the approach of a new tooth to the surface, rekindles the old trouble, to go once again through the same stages as before.

It is on the cheeks, the sides of the face, and the top of the head that these changes may be best studied, but there are other situations in which the same kind of process often goes on. It may be seen in the creases of the neck, or the folds of the thigh in fat children, only as two surfaces of skin are there in contact the fluid never dries to a crust, but the skin, red and sore and swollen, pours out an abundant secretion which, just as when it occurs behind the ears, gives out a strong and offensive smell. It occurs, too, at the bends of the joints, as under the knee, and at the inside of the elbow joint, as well as on the front of the chest, the back, and sometimes even over the whole body, and especially at any part where the pressure of the dress irritates the skin. When thus general, it seldom fails to pass into a chronic state such as to call for constant, skilled medical treatment.

The attack often comes on with general feverishness, a hot skin, fretfulness, and restlessness, which subside when the skin begins to discharge, though the discomfort produced by the local irritation still continues. At other times, and this perhaps more often when the eruption first appears on the head, its onset is more gradual, and slight scurfiness and redness at the top of the head are first noticed, and then a little crust forms there which is firmly adherent, and is, therefore, often not entirely removed as it should be, and thus bit by bit the mischief extends until its cure becomes tedious and troublesome. When either from neglect, or from the ailment having set in acutely, the affection of the scalp is severe, the child's state is one of much suffering. The whole of the scalp becomes hot and swollen, and covered over a large surface by a thick dirty crust, through cracks in which a thick ill-smelling greenish-yellow matter exudes on pressure. At different points around, pimples form with mattery heads,--pustules they are called--while the glands on each side of the neck become swollen and tender. When thus severe on the head it will be found also not merely on the face, but also on the body, and the poor suffering child is not only a miserable object to look upon, but, worn by constant restlessness, it loses flesh, and seems almost as though it could not long survive. Happily, however, the condition scarcely ever terminates fatally, though feeble health and stunted growth are not seldom the results of the early suffering. But besides, severe eczema in infancy always returns again and again in childhood and in after-life, and there is also a distinct connection between liability to eczema and to asthma; and this not simply nor mainly that the disappearance of an attack of eczema may be succeeded by an attack of asthma, but that the child who in infancy has had severe general eczema is more prone than another to develop a disposition to asthma as he attains the age of five or six, and this even though he should not have had any return of the skin affection in a severe form.

It is evident then, that one cannot take too much pains to guard against the occurrence of eczema if possible, and at any rate to prevent its becoming severe. The disposition to it is often controlled by very simple precautions, such as bathing the face, the moment the skin shows any redness or roughness, with thin gruel or barley water, then powdering it with starch powder, and when the infant goes out, smearing the spot very lightly with benzoated zinc ointment, and making the child wear a veil. It will be observed that the exclusion of the air is in all these cases the object of the application far more than any specific virtue which it is supposed to possess, and many of the worst cases of eczema in grown persons are treated, in the great hospital for skin diseases in Paris, by an india-rubber mask, or by india-rubber covering of the affected part, and benefit thereby without any medicated application whatever. The thin layer of scurf which often forms on an infant's head should not be allowed to remain there, since its presence is a source of irritation. If it is very adherent, the surface may be well greased overnight with a little clarified lard which will soften it, so that it can be readily washed off with weak soap and water in the morning. If, however, the skin is very irritable soap must not be used, but the head must be washed with yelk of egg and warm water, and instead of a sponge, which would be too harsh, it is better to employ a very large camel's hair brush or a soft shaving brush, which is more handy, and the surface after careful drying may be lightly smeared with zinc ointment. All ointments used must be washed off most scrupulously every day, otherwise they become rancid, irritate, and make matters worse.

When eczema sets in acutely, with general feverish disturbance, cooling medicines are required, and the help of the doctor becomes necessary. These are the cases in which the eruption is not confined to the head or the face, but extends over the body generally. The child must be dressed as loosely as possible; and when in its cot, should lie there with no other covering than its little shirt; and nothing gives so much relief to the irritation as the abundant use of powder, either simple starch powder, or ten parts of starch powder to one of oxide of zinc, or carbonate of bismuth. All powders must be absolutely free from grit, or, in other words, quite impalpable; otherwise they irritate the surface. On the face and other parts where it can be employed, the puff may be used to apply the powder; but between the creases of the skin--which it is important to keep apart--fine linen, lint, or charpie must be employed, covered freely with powder, so as to prevent the surfaces from coming into contact. If the irritation is very distressing, a weak spirit lotion with a little carbolic acid may sometimes be sponged over the surface, and the powder renewed immediately; or other forms of soothing lotions may be used to abate the irritation.

When the scalp is affected in the acute form of eczema crusts form very quickly; or in other cases they collect because people fear to disturb them when they see the raw surface beneath. It is, however, a grievous mistake to allow them to collect; they are in themselves a source of irritation, and they entirely prevent any application reaching the skin beneath. They must always be removed, and never be allowed to form again. They can be removed either by the employment of a poultice, half of bread, half of linseed meal, or by the application over-night of a handkerchief soaked in sweet oil, and covered over with a piece of oiled silk, which softens the crusts effectually, and allows of their easy removal by abundant washing with weak soap and water.

The best applications afterwards vary so much that it is impossible to lay down any positive rule. Sometimes the Carron oil, as it is termed: a liniment compound of equal parts of linseed oil and lime-water--a popular and most useful application in burns--gives most ease to the irritated skin; sometimes the mere exclusion of the air by means of the india-rubber cap; sometimes the abundant use of powder. In every case, at least once in every twenty-four hours the whole surface must be washed quite clean with barley water or thin gruel; and when the discharge lessens or ceases, as it will do in the course of time, then, but not till then, various ointments may be of service.

When the chronic stage arrives, in which the skin becomes dry and scaly, then is the time for tonics, for iron, sometimes for cod-liver oil, and for arsenic; of which latter remedy, however, the results are uncertain; while in the acute stage, its influence is simply mischievous. Nothing is more difficult, nor calls for more skill, or larger medical experience, than the proper management of the various forms of chronic eczema.

The question is sometimes asked whether it is safe to cure, or, as people call it, to dry up these eruptions in teething children. There can be no doubt but that it is very desirable to prevent their occurrence as far as may be by the use of the precautionary measures which I have explained. But when they have existed for some time, either attended with profuse discharge, or causing great irritation by their extent, there is no doubt but that care must be exercised in attempts at their cure, that soothing measures such as I have advocated should be chiefly employed, and that the sudden drying up of the discharge by a too abundant use of dusting powders must be avoided. If, too, the diminution of the rash were followed by a worsening of the child's condition, by feverishness, by heaviness of the head, or any sign of disturbance of the brain, the attempt to cure the rash must at once be abandoned. At the same time I must add that such occurrences are very rare, and that for one case where I have had to regret my success in curing the rash, I have seen fifty in which I have been mortified by the failure of my endeavour.

FOOTNOTES:

[8] The directions given by the distinguished chemist, Dr. Frankland, to whom I am indebted for the suggestion, are as follows: 'One-third of a pint of new milk is allowed to stand until the cream has settled; the latter is removed, and to the blue milk thus obtained about a square inch of rennet is to be added, and the milk vessel placed in warm water.' (I may add that the artificial rennet sold by most chemists may be substituted for the other.) 'In about five minutes the rennet, which may again be repeatedly used, being removed, the whey is carefully poured off, and immediately heated to boiling to prevent its becoming sour. A further quantity of curd separates, and must be removed by straining through calico. In one quarter of a pint of this hot whey is to be dissolved three-eighths of an ounce of milk sugar, and this solution, along with the cream removed from the one-third of a pint of milk, must be added to half a pint of new milk. This will constitute the food for an infant of from five to eight months old for twelve hours; or, more correctly speaking, it will be one-half of the quantity required for twenty-four hours. It

is absolutely necessary that a fresh quantity should be prepared every twelve hours; and it is scarcely necessary to add that the strictest cleanliness in all the vessels used is indispensable.'

[9] In our tables of mortality we find teething registered as having occasioned the death of nearly 5 (4.8) per cent. of all children who died in London under one year old; and of 7.3 per cent. of those who died between the age of twelve months and three years.

PART III.

ON THE DISORDERS AND DISEASES INCIDENT TO ALL PERIODS OF CHILDHOOD.

The ailments hitherto noticed are by no means all that may occur during infancy and early childhood, but those only which either happen then exclusively, or at least with far greater frequency than at other times.

It will be most convenient to consider the others under the different systems to which they belong, as diseases of the head, of the chest, and of the bowels.

Before entering on these new subjects, however, a few words may not be out of place with reference to what may be termed the second period of childhood. It is above all a time of wonderfully lessened sickness and mortality. We have not the means of stating exactly the rate at which mortality is lessened between the cessation of the first and the commencement of the second dentition; but we do know that it is ten times less between the age of one and five, and nearly twenty times less between five and ten than it was in the first year of existence.[10] A mother's anxiety then may safely be quieted after the first year of her infant's life, and still more after the first set of teeth have been cut, for if her child is strong and healthy then, there will be comparatively little to fear for its future.

Four years or thereabouts now follow, before any important change takes place in the child's condition, for it is not until between six and seven years old that the first set of teeth begin to be shed, and the second to take their place. This change of teeth too is of far less moment as far as the health is concerned, than was the cutting of the first set. The first dentition was the preparation for an entirely new mode of life for the child, and was intended to fit it for a life independent of its mother. The second has no such signification; it is a mere local alteration rendered necessary by the growth of the jaws, and takes place quietly, by the gradual absorption of the roots of the first set of teeth, brought about by the pressure of the others as they approach the surface. Four teeth in each jaw are new, and replace no others, but usually they are cut without much discomfort, and the wisdom teeth do not concern us here, for they do not appear until childhood has long passed.

But, though between the age of two years and of ten there is no important change, nor even preparation for a change in the constitution, the time is yet one of most active growth of the body, and consolidation of the skeleton. The stature increases from 2 ft. 6 in. to 4 ft. 6 in., and the weight nearly doubles, while at the same time the ends of the long bones previously connected with the shafts by means of cartilage or gristle, become firmly united by the conversion of that cartilage into bone, and a similar process goes on, though not completed till later, in the ribs and the breast bone.

Rapid increase of height and weight; conversion of the elements of bone into bone itself, formation of muscle out of the fat, which in the young child was stored up as so much building material for an edifice in course of construction, require for their accomplishment perfect health, and the power of converting to its highest purposes all the nourishment received. What wonder then, if from time to time, the machinery thus hardly taxed, fails to be quite equal to the demands upon it, if pains in the limbs--growing pains, as they are commonly called, or head-ache, tell of the inadequate nerve supply. Or if from the same cause, a vague feverish condition comes on, in which the temperature is slightly raised, and the child listless, and yet fretful, loses its cheerfulness, is dull at its easy tasks, and yet indifferent to play. This too is the time when any unsuspected defects, physical, or mental, or moral, begin to show themselves distinctly; when short sight becomes apparent so soon as the child has to learn its letters, when the dull hearing is perceived which makes it seem inattentive, and gives to its manner an unchildlike nervousness; and the weak intellect is displayed in causeless laughter, causeless mischief, causeless passion, imperfect power of articulation, or want of words, and by a restless busyness in doing nothing.

Of all these things I shall have to speak later on more fully. They are the things however, which only those mothers notice who live much with their children, who do not banish them all day long to the nursery or the school-room, and learn from another whether they fare well or ill. They and only they will notice these things in whom there dwells that which the poet tells us of:

The mother's love that grows From the soft child, to the strong man; now soft, Now strong as either, and still one sole same love.

FOOTNOTES:

[10] The exact numbers as given at p. xiv of the forty-fifth Report of the Registrar-General for all England in 1881 are to 1,000 living under one year 58 deaths; from one to five 6.1; from five to ten 3.3.

CHAPTER VI.

THE DISORDERS AND DISEASES OF THE BRAIN AND NERVOUS SYSTEM.

It is stated on good authority[11] that more than half of the deaths at all ages from these causes take place in children under five years, a fact which at first sight seems as inexplicable as it is startling. There is, however, a twofold explanation of it: the circulation through the much softer tissue of the brain, unenclosed within a firm bony case as in after-life, varies with far greater rapidity in the infant than in the grown person, and hence the organ is far more easily overfilled with or emptied of its blood. Besides, any organ in which growth is going on with great rapidity is proportionately liable to become disordered or diseased. Now the brain doubles its weight in the first two years of life, and attains nearly its full size by the end of the seventh year.

These two facts suggest a bright as well as a dark view of disorders of the brain and nervous system in early life. If disorder is more frequent, it is excited by slighter causes, is more likely to be temporary, and even its gravest symptoms, such as convulsions and paralysis, have a less serious import in the one case than in the others. If the grown man has a fit, and still more, if that fit is followed by paralysis, we fear and with reason that some vessel in the brain-substance has given way, or that some grave, probably irreparable damage has been inflicted on it. In the child, and especially in the young infant, these accidents may mean nothing more than that the brain has suddenly become over-filled with blood, or that it has been disturbed by irritation--I know of no better term--in some distant organ.

CONVULSIONS.--There are in the body two great nerve masses, the brain and the spinal cord, through which all parts are brought into relation with each other. The spinal cord or spinal marrow receives impressions from all parts, imparts movement to the limbs, as well as gives activity to the functions of the various internal organs. The brain is the controlling power, and governs more or less consciously the movements which the spinal cord originates, and hence in proportion as the development of the brain advances, and its controlling power increases, those involuntary movements, fits or convulsions, which originate in irritation of the spinal cord, become rarer. The brain, at the age of three years, is more than twice as large as in the first year of life, and deaths from convulsions have then sunk to a third of their former frequency; while from the age of ten to fifteen years, when the brain may be said to be perfected, only four per cent., instead of nearly eighty per cent. as in the first years of life, of all deaths from disorders of the nervous system are due to convulsions.[12]

I dwell on this subject the more because there is in a fit of convulsions something so intensely painful to behold that it is easy to exaggerate its danger, and to lose all presence of mind in panic. First, then, it is well to bear in mind that real disease of the brain rarely, very rarely, I do not say never, begins with convulsions; and next, that their real danger is in general in exactly opposite relation to the frequency of their occurrence. Convulsions now and then return thirty, forty, or more times in twenty-four hours, and continue to do so sometimes for three or four days together. They are, indeed, not without peril, for the perpetually returning disturbance of the circulation may give rise to an overfilling of the vessels of the brain, or to a stagnation of the blood within them, or the spasm may affect the muscles which open and close the entrance to the windpipe, and the child may die choked as in a paroxysm of whooping cough, or in a fit of spasmodic croup, or lastly the violent and frequently repeated muscular movements may at length exhaust its feeble frame. But still, such frequently recurring convulsions are in themselves no evidence that the brain is diseased; they do but show that the irritability of the spinal cord is increased to a degree which the brain is no longer able to control, and which therefore manifests itself in violent convulsive movements.

It is thus that the poison of scarlet fever or of small-pox sometimes displays its influence over the whole system by producing violent convulsions at the outset of those diseases; thus that they follow on some indigestible article of food, or that the mother, over-heated by violent exertion, or overwhelmed by the news of some unexpected calamity, sees her babe, to whom she is in the act of giving the breast, suddenly seized by a violent convulsion.

In every instance, therefore, the first business is to ascertain the cause of the convulsion, to determine the seat of the irritation which has excited the nervous system to such tumultuous reaction. The convulsion which ushers in any one of the eruptive fevers in the infant or in the child, is only an exaggeration of the shivering which precedes the onset of fever in the adult. Has the child been exposed to the contagion of measles, small-pox, or scarlatina? is it teething, and if so, when did its last tooth appear? of what did its last meal consist? when were its bowels last open? has it been exposed to the sun with its head uncovered? or has it, though in the shade, been sitting or playing out of doors in the intense heat of a summer's day? has it had a fall, or been frightened? or is it suffering from whooping-cough which has of late been very severe? or has its breathing been accompanied with a peculiar catch or crow, the sign of spasmodic croup, and have at the same time its hands been usually half clenched, and the thumb shut into the palm, the sign of that disturbance which at length has culminated in an attack of convulsions? Such are the questions, which in less time than it takes me to write, or others to read, the intelligent mother will put to herself, and will answer, instead of, in unreasoning alarm, giving all up as lost, or hastening without reflection to do something or other that were better left undone.

The first thing to do in every case of convulsions, be their cause what it may, is to loosen the dress, so that no string nor band may interfere with respiration, and for this purpose strings must be cut and dresses torn. The next thing is to dash cold water on the face to induce a deep inspiration, for sudden death in a fit almost always takes place from interruption to breathing. With the same purpose the forefinger should be put into the mouth, and run rapidly to the root of the tongue, which should be drawn forward. The object of doing this is twofold; first, to prevent the tongue falling back, as in these circumstances it is apt to do, over the entrance of the windpipe and so producing suffocation, and in the next place the act very frequently puts an end to the spasmodic closure of the windpipe, and is followed by a deep-drawn breath which announces the infant's safety. If the child has cut any teeth, the handle of a spoon, round which a bit of rag has been wrapped, or a bit of wood, or a thin strip of india-rubber, should be put between the teeth as far back as possible to prevent the tongue being bitten; and often this is all that can be done.

There are two circumstances, and two only, in which the warm bath is likely to be of use. At the onset of one of the eruptive fevers, a hot bath is sometimes of great service by stimulating the skin and thus bringing out the rash. In these cases the fit scarcely ever comes on in a child previously in perfect health, but for some hours at least it has appeared very ill, tossing about with great restlessness, with a dry, hot skin, and twitching of the tendons of the wrists; or, perhaps, with a pale face and cold hands and feet, but with the temperature of the body as high as 103° or 105° Here the hot bath at 96° to 98° even rendered more stimulating by the addition of mustard, and continued for not more than five minutes, is sometimes of great service, and is speedily followed by the cessation of the convulsions and the outbreak of the eruption.

These, too, are the cases in which the use of the wet sheet, as practised in hydropathic institutions, is sometimes of great benefit, but I do not advise its employment except under medical advice.

The second condition in which the bath, and here it is the tepid and not the hot bath--that is to say, the bath at from 87° to 90°-is of service, is where the child is feverish and restless from over-fatigue or over-excitement, or from exposure to the sun or to an excessively hot atmosphere, and convulsions have come on in the course of this ailing. Here the tepid bath for ten or fifteen minutes, coupled with the application of cold to the head, will soothe the excitement and prevent the return of the convulsions.

In neither this case, nor in that in which the hot bath is employed, is the result of the agent as magical as people sometimes seem to expect. It is rarely that convulsions cease while a child is actually in the bath. For the most part the influence of the bath is limited to abating their severity, shortening their duration, and indisposing to their return.

The bath, then, is to be used when either a stimulating or a soothing influence on the surface is likely to be of service, and only then. In cases where the fits are produced by constipation, by improper food, or by the irritation of a tooth pressing against the gum, it is idle to use it, and equally so in instances where many fits have been recurring in the course of the same day. Where that is the case it must be self-evident that, be the cause what it may, it must be one over which either a hot or a tepid bath can have no influence, and that, painful as it must be to wait a passive spectator, that position is far wiser than that of a mischievous meddler. It is some consolation, also, to know that unconsciousness to suffering attends convulsions.

There is one agent, chloroform, which often has a very remarkable influence in controlling frequently repeated convulsions. It is an agent, however, too hazardous to be trusted out of medical hands, and even when the doctor administers it himself, the parents must fully recognise the fact that, inasmuch as the child may die during a fit quite independently of breathing chloroform, so the occurrence of that catastrophe during its employment is not to be made a subject of self-reproach to them, or of blame to the doctor.

But you may ask whether there are no signs of that disturbance of the nervous system, by which you can judge beforehand that the occurrence of convulsions is probable. In proportion to the tender age of a babe, the greater is the probability, as I have already stated, that convulsions will be induced by slight causes, especially by such as digestive troubles. Unless you are aware of the phraseology that used at any rate to be common among nurses, you may be much alarmed at being told that the child who had seemed scarcely unwell has been very much convulsed, when all that is meant is that the child has shown some of the signs that threaten convulsions--has had, in short, what in the time of our grandmothers used to be called inward fits. A child thus affected lies as though it were asleep, winks its imperfectly closed eyes, and gently twitches the muscles of its face--a movement especially observable about the lips, which are drawn as though into a smile. Sometimes, too, this movement of the mouth is seen during sleep, and poets have told us that it is the angels' whisper which makes the babe to smile--I am sorry that its meaning in plain prose should be so different. If this condition increases, the child breathes with difficulty, its respiration sometimes seems for a moment almost stopped, and a livid ring surrounds the mouth. At every little noise the child wakes up; it makes a gentle moaning, brings up the milk while sleeping, or often passes a great quantity of wind, especially if the stomach is gently rubbed. When the disorder of the digestion, on whatever cause it depended, is removed, these symptoms speedily subside, nor is there much reason to fear general convulsions so long as no more serious symptoms show themselves. There is more cause for apprehension, however, when the thumbs are drawn into the palm, either habitually or during sleep; when the eyes are never more than half-closed during sleep; when the twitching of the muscles is no longer confined to the angles of the mouth, but affects the face and extremities; when the child awakes with a sudden start, its face growing flushed or livid, its eyes turning up under the upper eyelid, or the pupils suddenly dilating, while the countenance wears an expression of great anxiety or alarm, and the child either utters a shriek, or sometimes begins to cry.

When a fit comes on, the muscles of the face twitch, the body is stiff, immovable, and then in a short time, in a state of twitching motion, the head and neck are drawn backwards and the limbs violently bent and stretched. Sometimes these movements are confined to certain muscles or are limited to one side, and I may add that such cases are of more importance as far as the state of the brain is concerned than those in which the convulsions are general. The eye is fixed and does not see; the fingers may be passed over it without its winking, the pupil is immovably contracted or dilated; the ear is insensible even to loud sounds, the pulse is small, very frequent, often too small, and too frequent even for the skilled doctor to count it; the breathing hurried, laboured and irregular; the skin bathed in abundant perspiration.

After this condition has lasted for a minute, or ten minutes, or an hour or more, the convulsions cease; and the child either falls asleep, or lies for a short time as if it were bewildered, or bursts out crying, and then returns to its senses, or sinks into a state of stupor, in which it may either be perfectly motionless, or twitching of some muscles may still continue; or, lastly, it may, though this seldom happens, die in the fit.

It seems then, from all that has been said, that convulsions, though one of the most striking, are by no means one of the most conclusive signs of brain disease; that they are even more commonly the result of disorders of the nervous system from causes seated elsewhere, than of actual disease of what may be termed the great nervous centre.

We may now therefore pass to the examination of these diseases, which for the purposes of this book may be considered under the two heads of congestion and inflammation.

I am forced to use these terms in somewhat of a popular sense, for to attempt in a little book like this to define everything with strict scientific accuracy would simply confuse and mislead.

CONGESTION OF THE BRAIN.--By congestion of the brain is meant a condition in which its vessels are overcharged with blood; a condition which if it exists in an aggravated degree, ends either in the pouring out of blood on, or into the brain, on the one hand, or in inflammation on the other. Either of these terminations, however, is so rare in the previous healthy child, that I shall confine my remarks entirely to congestion of the brain, an affection specially liable to occur in children during teething. A certain degree of feverishness almost always accompanies teething. It is, therefore, not difficult to understand how, when the circulation is in a state of permanent excitement, a very slight cause may suffice to overturn its equilibrium, and occasion a greater flow of blood to the brain than the organ is able to bear. Congestion of the brain, however, is not by any means limited to this season, but may occur at other times without any obvious exciting cause, and with no other explanation than is furnished by the well-known fact that all periods of development such as childhood, are periods during which the growing organs are most apt to become disordered.

In the great majority of cases the symptoms of congestion of the brain come on slowly; and for the most part, general uneasiness, or disordered state of the bowels, which are usually, though not invariably constipated, and feverishness precede for a few days the more serious attack. The head by degrees becomes hot, the child grows restless and fretful, and seems distressed by light, or noise, or sudden motion, and children who are old enough sometimes complain of their head. Usually too, vomiting occurs repeatedly; a symptom of the greatest importance, since it may exist before there is any well-marked sign of head affection. Causeless frequently repeated vomiting in a child not ill but ailing, is nine times out of ten a sign of mischief in the head. The degree of fever which attends this condition varies much, and its returns are irregular; but any one who knows how to feel the pulse will find it permanently quickened, and if the head is unclosed the pulsations of the brain may be seen and felt distinctly. The sleep is disturbed, the child often waking with a start, while there is occasional twitching of the muscles of its face, or of the tendons of its wrist.

The child may continue in this condition for many days and then recover its health without any medical interference. This is especially likely to be the case with children while teething, the fever subsiding, the head growing cool, and the little one appearing quite well so soon as the tooth has cut through the gum, but the approach of each tooth to the surface being attended by the recurrence of the same symptoms.

The fortunate issue of these cases though frequent, is by no means invariable, for sometimes they are but the precursors of that formidable, I might indeed say, all but hopeless disease, water on the brain. But even of itself congestion of the brain is by no means a trivial ailment, for it may pass into a stage in which the smaller discomforts of the child lead to the sad mistake that the condition of the child is improving, instead of which it is really the dulling of sensibility from approaching death. The head, indeed, becomes less hot, the flush of the face grows slighter and less constant; but the countenance is heavy and anxious, the indifference to surrounding objects increases, and the child lies in a state of torpor or drowsiness, from which indeed it can at first be roused to complete consciousness The manner on being roused is always fretful, but, if old enough to talk, the child's answers are natural, though generally very short; and murmuring, 'I am so sleepy, so sleepy,' it subsides into its former drowsiness. The bowels generally continue constipated, and the vomiting seldom ceases, though it is sometimes less frequent than before. In this state, without any apparent cause, the child sometimes has an attack of convulsions, which subsiding, leaves the torpor deeper than before. The fits return, and death may take place in one of them, or the torpor growing more profound after each convulsive seizure, the child at length dies insensible.

Now and then, especially in infants of only five or six months old, recovery takes place even where there seemed almost no ground for hope. The overfull vessels have at length relieved themselves, fluid has been poured out into the cavities of the brain, the yielding skull has given way under the pressure from within, and should the child after all survive, its large head, due to chronic water on the brain, tells to all who know how to interpret the signs, the tale of its past illness, and the manner of its imperfect recovery.

Cases such as these are obviously beyond the reach of domestic management, and call for all the resources of medical skill. The mistake commonly made is that of calling in the doctor too late, because it is not realised how grave may be the import of symptoms which at first appear so little alarming; and the so-called experienced nurse having said, 'Oh! it's nothing but the baby's teeth,' time is lost and danger not anticipated till too late for remedy.

The application of two, three, or four leeches at the very outset of these cases is often of great service, and sometimes cuts short symptoms which had seemed very threatening. The doctor, of course, must be the judge of its expediency, but I refer to it because I have known parents raise objections to it, and beg to have milder means tried first. It must be borne in mind then, that whenever leeches are of use it is at the beginning of an attack, and that the opportunity once let slip does not return. Purgatives, cold to the head, saline medicines, and perhaps some carefully selected sedative, are the measures which will probably be employed in most cases, but success will in great measure depend on the minute care with which all the details which I dwelt on in the introduction, are carried out.

It is not always, indeed, that active treatment is desirable, and gentle measures then suffice; but nothing except close and frequent watching can enable the doctor to steer safely between the two opposite dangers of too little and too much.

When I come to speak of the eruptive fevers, I shall have to mention the convulsions and other signs of most serious brain disturbance, which sometimes occur at their outset, and which are due to the condition of the blood charged with the fever poison.

A somewhat similar set of symptoms, attributed with reason to the overheated state of the blood, occurs in cases of sunstroke. It is true that sunstroke, with the formidable characters that it presents in hot countries, is not seen in England, but even here the mere exposure of an infant or young child to an overheated atmosphere, is by no means unattended with risk, and I refer to it here, because mothers are by no means aware of the danger, and believe that it suffices to guard the child from the direct rays of the sun.

Alarm, restlessness, and fretfulness, alternating with drowsiness, hurried, irregular breathing, intense heat of skin, violent beating of the open part of the head, twitching of the limbs, and starting of the tendons of the wrists, with a pulse too rapid to be counted, are the symptoms when the attack is severe. Convulsions are rare, though they sometimes occur. Sickness is almost invariable, the stomach rejecting everything, and the bowels are almost invariably relaxed, severe diarrh[oe]a or dysentery sometimes coming on, as the brain disturbance abates. The first shock may kill the child in a few hours, or it may sink under the subsequent diarrh[oe]a, but as a rule recovery eventually takes place.

All cases, indeed, are not equally severe, but all require careful and gentle treatment, the cool and darkened room, the quiet, the cold to the head, the tepid bath, and on the part of everyone the care not to allow the apparently serious condition of the child to urge them to those active measures which will here be out of place, and destroy the hopes which would revive after a few hours of patience and gentle means.

Really acute inflammation of the brain is of so rare occurrence except as the result of accident or injury, and its symptoms are of so serious a character, even from the first, that medical advice is obviously needed at once. I shall, therefore, pass it over here, and endeavour to describe two forms of inflammation of the brain which are much more frequent, and at their commencement more likely to be overlooked.

=Water on the Brain.=--One of these is the form of inflammation commonly known as water on the brain, a term which, though incorrect medically, has the advantage of being well understood. This, now, is not a simple disease, occurring in a previously healthy child, but it is a disease dependent on the same state of constitution as gives rise in other children to consumption, or scrofula, or disease of the mesenteric glands.

It is this circumstance which renders the disease so serious, and recovery from it so extremely rare. This it is also which makes it so desirable to become acquainted with its symptoms, both that you may be alive to the approach of danger, and also not indulge in needless alarm when brain symptoms occur from other causes which have no relation whatever to those which give rise to water on the brain.

The disease comparatively seldom comes on in a child who had previously seemed in perfect health; a state of vague ailing usually precedes its outbreak. The child loses flesh and strength, and the look of health, and the lustre of the eye, and the silky softness of the hair. The appetite becomes uncertain, the bowels irregular, with a tendency to constipation; there are little feverish attacks for a few hours, subsiding of their own accord. The sleep is not sound, the temper uncertain, the child tires even of its favourite toys; the brightness of the little face is changed for a strange, weird, wistful look--an unnatural earnestness; the child sits for moments gazing upward on vacancy, as though it saw, or sought something beyond.

By degrees these vague premonitions, which may continue for weeks, become more and more marked till they pass into what may be called the first stage of the affection, in which there are signs of congestion of the brain, such as I have already described, coupled with general irregular attacks of feverishness. The child becomes more gloomy, more pettish, and slower in its movements, and is little pleased by its usual amusements. Or, at other times, its spirits are very variable; it will sometimes cease suddenly in the midst of its play, and run to hide its head in its mother's lap, putting its hands to its head, and complaining of headache, or saying merely that it is tired and sleepy, and wants to go to bed. Sometimes, too, it will turn dizzy, as you will know, not so much from its complaint of dizziness as from its suddenly standing still, gazing around for a moment as if lost, and then either beginning to cry at the strange sensation, or seeming to awake from a reverie, and at once returning to its play. The infant in its nurse's arms betrays the same sensation by a sudden look of alarm, a momentary cry, and a hasty clinging to its nurse. If the child can walk it may be observed to drag one leg, halting in its gait, though but slightly, and seldom as much at one time as at another, so that both the parents and the medical attendant may be disposed to attribute it to an ungainly habit which the child has contracted. The appetite is usually bad, though sometimes very variable; and the child, when apparently busy at play, may all at once throw down its toys and beg for food, then refuse what is offered; or taking a hasty bite may seem to nauseate the half-tasted morsel, may open its mouth, stretch out its tongue, and heave as if about to vomit. The thirst is seldom considerable, and sometimes there is an actual aversion to drink as well as to food, apparently from its exciting or increasing the sickness. The stomach, however, seldom rejects everything; but the same food as occasions sickness at one time is retained at another. Sometimes the child vomits only after taking food, at other times, even when the stomach is empty, it brings up some greenish phlegm without much effort, and with no relief. These attacks of vomiting seldom occur oftener than two or three times a day, but they may return for several days together, the child's head probably growing heavier, and its headache more severe. The bowels during this time are disordered, generally constipated from the very first, though their condition in this respect sometimes varies at the commencement of the disease. The evacuations are usually scanty, sometimes pale, often of different colours, almost always deficient in bile, frequently mud-coloured and very offensive. The tongue is not dry, generally rather red at the tip and edges, coated with white fur in the centre and yellowish towards the root, but occasionally very moist, and uniformly coated with white fur. The skin is harsh, but not very hot, the temperature seldom above 100?Fahr., varying causelessly, but usually higher towards evening than in the daytime. The nostrils are dry, the eyes lustreless, and the child sheds no tears. It is drowsy, and will sometimes want to be put to bed two or three times in a day; but it is restless, sleeps ill, grinds its teeth in sleep, lies with its eyes partially open, awakes with the slightest noise, or even starts up in alarm without any apparent cause. At night, too, the existence of intolerance of light is often first noticed in consequence of the child's complaints about the presence of the candle in the room.

I have purposely dwelt long on this preliminary stage because it is only in it that treatment is likely to be of any service, while the very indefiniteness of the symptoms constantly leads to their being overlooked, or referred to teething, or thought at any rate to be a mere temporary ailment for which it is not worth while to call in the doctor.

After four or five days, however, the illness of the child becomes too marked to escape notice. All cheerfulness has fled, the eyes are closed to shut out the light, the child lies apparently dozing, but answers questions rationally, in a short quick manner in as few words as possible, and from time to time complains of its head, or utters a short, sharp lamentable cry. The night brings with it no other change than an increase of restlessness, attended sometimes with noisy cries, or with the wandering talk of delirium. Sickness often diminishes, but the bowels continue constipated, and it is to be noted that whereas in fevers the bowels are distended with wind, here all wind has disappeared and the belly is sunken to a striking degree.

Next comes the last stage. Each stage is distinguished by peculiarities of the pulse which tell the expert what is passing; quick and regular in the first stage; irregular and slower in the second; quick, variable, irregular from time to time in the third; growing more rapid and more feeble as the end arrives. Squinting, stupor, dilated pupil, difficulty of swallowing, tremulous limbs, convulsions, profound insensibility, such are the series of occurrences which bring on death usually within a fortnight, always within three weeks from the appearance of the first decided symptoms.

What are you to do in these cases? Above all save yourselves the heartbreak of feeling that you have overlooked the premonitory symptoms of the disease. Guard with special care the health of any child in whose family a disposition to consumptive disease has ever shown itself, and keep it at any cost from the risk of catching the hooping cough or measles. Since, too, it is not in early infancy, but after the age of one year, and in the majority of instances between the ages of three and six years that this disease occurs, that is to say, at the time when the brain begins to be most actively exercised, when the new world on which the child is just entering brings with it new wonders every day; be very careful not to over-stimulate its intelligence, over-excite its imagination, or over-strain its mental powers. After the age of ten the great danger is over; up to that time it is the health of the body which requires care; not fuss, not rearing like a hothouse plant, but the healthy training that may fortify the system.

When any signs such as I have described indicate the threatening of disease, do not look on them as within the scope of domestic management, but place the child at once under the watchful care of a skilful doctor. I have seen but one recovery in all my life, after the disease had fully set in, and that was a recovery almost worse than death.

=Earache.=--There is another form of inflammation of the brain which is likewise oftenest met with in children who are of weakly constitution, or of scrofulous habit, or in whom scarlet fever has left behind that very troublesome ailment, discharge from the ear. This is so tedious, so difficult to cure, so apt to return under the influence of very slight causes, that people are too ready to put up with it as an inconvenience which it is useless to try to remedy.

In addition, however, to the risk of the child's hearing being impaired by the extension of the mischief to the internal ear, there is another still greater danger, namely, that of the disease passing from the ear to the brain, and producing inflammation of its membranes, or even abscess of its substance.

It is therefore of the greatest moment that every case of chronic discharge from the ear should be looked on as important, and that no pains be spared to bring about its cure; and further, that during its continuance the slightest sign of disturbance of the brain--headache, sickness, feverishness, and dulness--should at once be noticed, and the advice of a competent doctor be immediately sought for.

These dangers, however, follow almost entirely on long-continued discharges from the ear, but do not attend that acute inflammation of the passage to the ear which is often met with in childhood, and the symptoms of which sometimes cause needless fear, from being taken for those of inflammation of the brain. Attacks of earache are most frequent before the first set of teeth have been cut, and are by no means rare in young children, who are perfectly unable to point out the seat of their sufferings. The attack sometimes comes on quite suddenly, but usually the child is languid and fretful for a period varying from a few hours to one or two days before acute pain is experienced. In this premonitory stage, however, it will often cry if tossed or moved briskly; noise seems unpleasant to it, and it does not care to be played with; while children who are still at the breast show a disinclination to suck, though they will take food from a spoon. The infant seeks to rest its head on its mother's shoulder, or, if lying in its cot, moves its head uneasily from side to side, and then buries its face in the pillow. If you watch closely, you will see that it is always the same side of the head which it seeks to bury in the pillow, or to rest on its nurse's arm, and that no other position seems to give any ease, except this one, which, after much restlessness, the child will take up, and to which, if disturbed, it will always return. The gentle support to the ear seems to soothe the little patient: it cries itself to sleep, but after a short doze, some fresh twinge of pain arouses it, or some accidental movement disturbs it, and it awakes crying aloud, and refusing to be pacified, and may continue so for hours together. Sometimes the ear is red, and the hand is often put to the affected side of the head, but neither of these symptoms is constant. The intensity of the pain seldom lasts for more than a few hours, when, in many instances a copious discharge of matter takes place from the ear, and the child is well. In some instances, indeed, the subsidence of the disease on one side is followed by a similar attack on the opposite side, and the same acute suffering is once more gone through, and terminates in the same manner. Sometimes, too, this complete cure does not take place, but the earache abates, or altogether ceases, for a day or two, and then returns; no discharge, or but a very scanty discharge, taking place, while, for weeks together, the child has but few intervals of perfect ease. In infants, earache seldom follows this chronic course, but it does sometimes in older children, and is then of the more importance, since it shows that the disease is no longer confined to the external passage, but has extended to the internal ear.

In children who are too young to express their sufferings by words, the violence of their cries, coupled with the absence of any sign of disease in the chest or the bowels, naturally leads to the suspicion of something being wrong in the head. There are several facts, however, which may satisfy you that the case is not one of water on the brain--the child does not vomit, its bowels are not constipated, there is but little fever, the cries are loud and passionate, and are attended with shedding tears. If you watch closely, you will notice the dread of movement and the evident relief afforded by resting one side of the head, and always the same side, while often the movement of the hand to the head, and the redness of the ear, with the swelling at its entrance, will all serve to point to that organ as the source of the trouble. Sometimes, when in doubt, you will be able to satisfy yourselves that the cause of the suffering is in the ear by pressing the gristle of the organ slightly inwards, which will produce very evident pain on the affected side, while on the other side it will not occasion any suffering.

The treatment of this painful affection is very simple. In many instances the suffering is greatly relieved by warm fomentations, or by applying to the ear a poultice of hot bran or camomile flowers, while at the same time a little warm oil and laudanum are dropped into the ear. When these means do not bring relief, a leech applied on the bone directly behind the ear seldom fails to give ease; while the disposition to the frequent return of the attack is often controlled by a series of small blisters, not larger than a sixpence, behind the ear. As soon as the tendency has sufficiently abated to admit of it, the ear should be syringed out twice a day with warm water, or with equal parts of warm water and Goulard lotion; but if pain or discharge still continues, medical advice must in all cases be sought for.

=Chronic Water on the Brain.=--There is still another form of inflammation of the brain, concerning which a few words will suffice. It constitutes what is termed chronic water on the brain, and in this instance the term is a correct one, for the disease usually depends on a slow form of inflammation of the lining membrane of the cavities of the brain, often beginning before, still oftener very soon after, birth, which ends in the pouring out of a quantity of fluid into them sufficient to enlarge the head to three or four times its natural dimensions.

Such cases are very sad and very hopeless, and the great resource, which is sometimes adopted by medical men, of puncturing the head and letting out the fluid, is very seldom successful.

But there are more hopeful cases sometimes met with, those namely of children in whom, either from simple weakness, or from that constitutional disorder called rickets, bone formation has been backward, and the head has consequently long remained unclosed. If such children, either from the irritation of teething, or from the straining during paroxysms of hooping cough, suffer from congestion of the brain, fluid may be poured out, which, not being compressed by the too yielding skull, may in consequence enlarge it. These cases, however, may be distinguished from the other more serious ones by the date of their commencement, which is always much later than that of the other form, by the symptoms which attend them being less severe, and by the enlargement of the skull being far slighter.

Still they require watching, for while with improved health the enlargement ceases, the fluid is in a measure absorbed, and the head diminishes in size, though always remaining larger than the average; brain mischief is yet more readily set up in children with such antecedents than in others.

The anxiety of parents about the size or shape of their child's head after infancy has passed, is perfectly needless. When the head has once closed it always remains so. An odd shape, with an unusual protuberance of the forehead and the hind head, sometimes remain as the evidence of that condition in infancy to which I have just referred. It is, however, an evidence of mischief passed, not of mischief going on. In children too who have suffered from rickets, an affection rarely met with except among the poor in crowded cities, distortion of the limbs is often associated with a peculiar form of the skull, but in this too there is nothing to call for anxiety, still less to excite alarm. It is only a preternaturally small head and shelving forehead, which are found associated with mental deficiency; otherwise the greatest varieties of size and shape, of symmetry, or of want of it, may be associated with an equal variety of intellectual endowment, which is just as likely to be above as below the average.

=Brain Disorder from Exhaustion.=--It may at first sight appear strange that before leaving the subject of congestion and inflammation of the brain, I should find it necessary to give a caution against being misled by symptoms which though in some respects similar to those of congestion or inflammation, are in reality due to an exactly opposite condition.

This mistake, however, is very possible; doctors themselves sometimes fall into it, and some distinguished physicians have thought it worth their while to lay down very minute rules for distinguishing between the two opposite states. Headache we all know attends an overfull condition of the vessels of the brain, and grown persons usually suffer from it severely before an attack of apoplexy; but we also know that bad headache accompanies states of great weakness, and that it is one of the most distressing consequences from which a woman suffers who has lost much blood in her confinement. In just the same way, the infant who has been exhausted by diarrh[oe]a or by some trying illness, or who after weaning has been kept on a diet not sufficiently nutritious, may show symptoms of disorder of the brain.

It may become irritable, restless, very startlish, with occasional flushings of the face, moaning in its sleep, and sleeping with half-closed eyes. But the head is not hotter than the rest of the body; if the head is not closed, the open part or fontanelle is not tense and pulsating, but flat or even depressed, the hands and feet are cool, and very readily become cold; there may be occasional vomiting, but nothing like the constant sickness of real brain-disease, the bowels are not shrunken but distended, constipation is not present, but on the contrary there is a disposition to diarrh[oe]a. If the symptoms are misinterpreted and wrongly treated, unmistakable signs of exhaustion at last come on, and the child may die from its not being borne in mind that results at first sight much the same may flow from causes diametrically opposite.

The moral of this is too obvious for me to need insist upon it. Cold to the head, low diet, aperients, possibly leeches, are needed in the one case; increased nourishment, perhaps stimulants, in the other. In every instance where symptoms of brain disorder occur in the child, remember the grievous consequences of a mistake as to their nature, and seek for further help and guidance to preserve you from the possibility of error.

=Spasmodic Croup.=--I have already tried to explain how, in early life, the brain is often unequal to control the sensitiveness of the nervous system to various sources of irritation from without, and how, in consequence this irritation manifests itself by those involuntary movements which we call convulsions. But in addition to, or in the place of those violent contortions or convulsions, the same condition shows itself sometimes in disordered action of the muscles which subserve parts not directly subject to the will, as those for instance which open and close the entrance to the windpipe, or glottis as it is called in medical phraseology.

Cases in which this occurs are known in popular language as child-crowing, or spasmodic croup, from the peculiar catch or crow which accompanies the entrance of air through the spasmodically contracted opening of the windpipe; a spasm which if severe and sufficiently continued closes the opening altogether, so that after fruitless efforts to get its breath the child dies suffocated. This affection occurs chiefly during teething, just as the fits of a hysterical girl oftenest occur during the transition from girlhood to womanhood; but many other causes besides the local irritation of the teeth may produce it, such as constipation, indigestible food, or disorder of the bowels.

It does not often occur in perfectly healthy children; but an infant who is attacked by it is usually observed to have been drooping for some time previously, to have lost its appetite, to have become fretful by day and restless at night, and to present many of those ill-defined ailments which are popularly ascribed to teething. At length, after these symptoms have lasted for a few days or weeks, a slight crowing sound is occasionally heard with the child's respiration, shorter, more high-pitched, but less loud than the hoop of hooping cough. Usually it is first noticed on the child awaking out of sleep, but sometimes it is perceived during a fit of crying, or comes on while the infant is sucking. The spasm may have been excited by some temporary cause, and the sound which is its token may not be heard again; but generally it returns after the lapse of a few hours, or of a day or two, and its loudness usually increases in proportion as its return becomes more frequent. It will soon be found that certain conditions favour its occurrence; that the child wakes suddenly with an attack of it, that excitement induces it, or the act of swallowing, or the effort at sucking, so that the child will drop the nipple, make a peculiar croupy sound with its breathing, and then return to the breast again. Throughout the whole course of the affection, its attacks will be found to be more frequent by night than by day; and to occur mostly soon after the child has lain down to sleep, or towards midnight, when the first sound sleep is drawing to a close.

At first, the child seems, during the intervals of the attack, much as before; except, perhaps, that it is rather more pettish and wilful; but it is not long before graver symptoms than the occasional occurrence of an unusual sound when the child draws a deep breath excite attention, and give rise to alarm. Fits of difficult breathing occasionally come on, in which the child throws its head back, while its face and lips become livid, or an ashy paleness surrounds the mouth, slight convulsive movements pass over the muscles of the face; the chest is motionless, and suffocation seems impending. But in a few seconds the spasm yields, expiration is effected, and a long loud crowing inspiration succeeds, or the child begins to cry. Breathing now goes on naturally: the crowing is not repeated, or the crying ceases; a look of apprehension dwells for a moment on the infant's features, but then passes away; it turns once more to its playthings, or begins sucking again as if nothing were the matter. A few hours, or even a few days, may pass before this alarming occurrence is again observed, but it does recur, and another symptom of the disturbance of the nervous system is soon superadded, if it has not, as is often the case, existed from the very beginning. This consists in a peculiar contraction of the hands and feet; a state which may likewise not infrequently be noticed during infancy, unattended by any peculiarity in breathing. It differs much in degree; sometimes the thumb is simply drawn into the palm while the fingers are unaffected; at other times the fingers are closed more or less firmly, and the thumb is shut into the palm; or, coupled with this, the hand itself is forcibly flexed on the wrist. In the slightest degree of affection of the foot, the great toe is drawn a little away from the other toes; in severer degrees the toe is drawn away still further, and the whole foot is forcibly bent upon the ankle, and its sole directed a little inwards. Affection of the hands generally precedes the affection of the feet, and may even exist without it, but the spasmodic contraction of the feet never exists without the hands being involved likewise. At first this state is temporary, but it does not come on and cease simultaneously with the attacks of crowing breathing, though generally much aggravated during its paroxysms. Sometimes a child in whom the crowing breathing has been heard, will awake in the morning with the hands and feet firmly bent, though he may not have had any attack of difficult breathing during the night. When the contraction is but slight, children still use their hands; but when considerable they cannot employ them, and they sometimes cry, as if the contraction of the muscles were attended with pain. Sometimes, too, there is a degree of puffiness both of hands and feet, a sort of dropsical condition, which, whenever it is present, adds much to the anxiety with reference to the child.

As the condition becomes more serious, a slight crowing sound is heard each time the child draws its breath, the fits of difficult breathing are much more severe; they last longer, and sometimes end in general convulsions. The breathing now does not return at once to its natural frequency, but continues hurried for a few minutes after the occurrence of each fit of difficult breathing, and is sometimes attended with a little wheezing. The slightest cause is now sufficient to bring on an attack; it may be produced by a current of air, by a sudden change of temperature, by slight pressure on the windpipe, by the act of swallowing, or by momentary excitement. The state of sleep seems particularly favourable to its occurrence, and the short fitful dozes are interrupted by the return of impending suffocation, in one paroxysm of which longer and severer than the others the infant may fall back dead.

It scarcely need be said that the great majority of cases have no such sad ending as I have described, but still, whenever this spasm exists, even in a slight degree, there is always the possibility, never to be forgotten, of a sudden catastrophe. Usually, after some tooth has been cut which caused special irritation, or as disorder of the bowels has been set right, the symptoms abate by degrees, and then cease altogether, though liable to be reproduced by the same causes as those to which they were originally due.

The seeking out and removing the exciting causes must be the care of the medical man, but there are some special precautions which come within the mother's own province to observe.

First of all, as sudden excitement, and especially a fit of crying, are likely to bring on the attack, and since there is a possibility that any attack may prove fatal, the greatest care must be taken in the management of the child to avoid all unnecessary occasion of annoyance or of distress.

Although the benefit that accrues from fresh air, or from a change of air, is often very great, yet it is very important that the child should not be exposed to the cold or wind, for I have seen such exposure followed by a severe attack of difficult breathing, or by the occurrence of general convulsions. Another reason for caution in this respect is that the occurrence of catarrh is almost sure to be followed by an aggravation of the spasmodic affection, which, though previously slight, may thereby be rendered serious or even dangerous.

I have nothing to add to what I have already said with reference to the treatment of the attack, when actual convulsions come on. Since, however, in this affection convulsions may occur quite unexpectedly at any moment, it is well always to have a basin of cold water and a bunch of feathers handy, in order to be able at once to dash the water on the child's face, and induce that deep inspiration which saves it from the threatening danger. If this should not suffice, the finger must be put into the mouth, and run over the back of the tongue in the way that I have already explained when speaking of convulsions. Now and then it happens, though but very rarely, that violent general convulsions come on in infancy quite independent of spasmodic croup, not preceded nor attended by any sign of disease of the brain, and which end in the course of some hours or of a few days in death, the child being partly worn out by the violence of the muscular movements, partly by the disturbance of breathing which each fit occasions. Happily, however, in most of these instances the convulsions by degrees lessen both in violence and frequency, and the child recovers.

=Epilepsy.=--There is one other point of view from which convulsions in infancy and early childhood must be looked on with apprehension, and that is from their being frequently followed in after years by epilepsy. In nearly a fifth of all cases of epilepsy in childhood that have come under my notice the first occurrence of fits dated back to early infancy, and this, even though an interval of years had passed between the last fit in infancy and the first in childhood. It seems, indeed, as though there were in these cases a peculiar abiding sensitiveness of the nervous system, which, dating back from very early life, dependent often on hereditary predisposition, was kindled into activity by any special cause, such as the cutting of the second set of teeth, or the transition from boyhood or girlhood to manhood or womanhood.

In the child, just as in the grown person, epilepsy manifests itself in two different ways; either by momentary unconsciousness, or by violent convulsions, in which latter there is little distinction from the occasional fit which may be observed at any period of infancy.

The attacks of momentary unconsciousness often pass long unnoticed. They occur, perhaps, when the child is at play or at meals; it stops as if dazed, its eye fixed on vacancy; if standing, it does not fall, nor does it drop the toy or the spoon which it was holding from its hand. If speaking, it just breaks off in the midst of the half-uttered sentence. Then, in less time than it takes to tell, it suddenly looks up again, finishes what it was saying, or goes on with its play, or with its meal as though nothing had happened; or it suffices to call the child and the cloud passes from its face, and it is itself again; and the nurse or perhaps even the mother, thinks that it is some odd trick which the child has got. By degrees the attacks become more frequent, and may continue to recur several times a day without any obvious cause, even for months; and this without any change in their character. By degrees, however, under their influence, an alteration takes place slowly in the child's disposition. It loses its cheerfulness and brightness, its face assumes a heavy look, it becomes fretful, and its intelligence grows duller.

Almost invariably after the attacks of this, which has been called the petit mal, have continued for some months, a change begins to take place, which does not fail to excite attention and to cause alarm. If seated, the child's head drops forward for a moment, and strikes against the table; if standing, it becomes for an instant dizzy, and staggers, or even falls, and then there is twitching of one limb, or of the muscles of the face, and then the complete fit of epilepsy, ushered in sometimes, but not always, by a momentary cry, and then the convulsive twitching of one limb, followed in a minute or in less time by convulsions of the whole body as well as of the limbs. The upturned eyes, which do not see, are horribly distorted, the child foams at the mouth, it is insensible, and the insensibility deepens into stupor, or is followed by heavy sleep, for a quarter of an hour, or an hour or more, from which the patient arouses feeling tired and bruised, and often with an aching head, but with no remembrance of what has passed during the seizure so distressing to bystanders.

It has throughout been my endeavour not to lose sight of those for whom this little book has been written, and with reference to epilepsy, as with reference to many other things, I pass over much that would be important to the practitioner of medicine, to dwell on those points which mainly interest the parents, and which they are perfectly able to appreciate.

The question is often put as to the probability of fits terminating in epilepsy; or, on the other hand, as to the ground for hope in any case that epileptic attacks, which have already often recurred, will eventually cease. In the first place, no conclusion can safely be drawn from the severity of a convulsion, nor from its general character, as to the probability of its frequent recurrence, or of its passing into permanent epilepsy. The severity of a fit certainly affords no reason for this apprehension, nor does its recurrence, so long as a distinct exciting cause can be discovered for each return. The fits, which cease in the teething child when the gum is lanced, and which, on each succeeding return are equally relieved by the same proceeding, do not imply that there is any great tendency on their part to become habitual. In the same way, the attacks which follow on constipation, or on indigestion, or on some other definite exciting cause, may probably with care be guarded against, and their return prevented. It is not the violence of a single fit, nor even the frequent return of fits for a limited time, which warrants the gravest apprehension; but it is their recurrence when all observable causes of irritation have passed away; it is their return when the child is otherwise apparently in perfect health.

If, on the one hand, the violence of a convulsion does not by any means imply the greater proportionate risk of its recurrence, so neither can any hopeful conclusion be drawn from the slightness of an attack, or from its momentary duration. In childhood, such attacks are at least as common preludes to confirmed epilepsy as in the adult, and are the more deserving of attention from their very liability to be overlooked. I believe, too, that an imperfect suspension of consciousness, the child knowing what passes, though unable to speak, is not very uncommon, and further, that it is far from unusual to have the early stage of epilepsy in childhood announced by sudden incoherent talking for a few seconds, or by a wild look; a cry of surprise, or a short fit of sobbing, announcing as in a hysterical girl, the close of the paroxysm. The early symptoms of epilepsy in childhood are also the more likely to be misinterpreted from the circumstance that they are frequently accompanied by a moral perversion much more striking than any loss of mental power. It is true that in early life there are alternations of intellectual activity and mental indolence, of quickness and comparative dulness, which all who have had much to do with education are well aware of, and which are perfectly compatible with health of body and health of mind. But changes in the moral character of a child who is still under the same influences, have a far deeper meaning than is often attached to them; a child does not suddenly become wayward, fretful, passionate, or mischievous, except under the pressure of some grave cause.

One other point there is also to be borne in mind; namely, that the child is compelled by the vague sensation of hitherto unknown dread, not to conceal the early symptoms of epilepsy as the grown person would do; longing as the child does for love and sympathy, and weakened in its moral force, it craves for more love, more sympathy, it exaggerates its symptoms, it assumes some which do not exist at all. The conclusion is a natural one, but none the less mistaken, that the child who is discovered to be shamming has nothing the matter with it--is simply a naughty child. This is a fact of much importance, on which I shall have occasion to insist further on.

In the child, as in the adult, epilepsy blunts the intellect as well as weakens the moral powers; and does both more speedily and more effectually in proportion as the child is younger, and its mind and will are less developed. And yet this has its compensation; for as the powers fade quickly, so, if the attacks cease, they recover with surprising rapidity, and as the moral powers are the first to suffer, so they are the first to regain--I will not say full vigour, but at least a degree which raises the children to be objects of specially tender affection, rather than of pity and compassion.

The conditions which justify the most hopeful view of any case of epilepsy are then, first, the absence of any history of frequently recurring convulsions in early infancy; secondly, the existence of a distinct exciting cause for the attacks; thirdly, the rarity of their return far more than their slight severity; and lastly, the more the attacks approach in character to what one knows as hysteria, the less profound the insensibility in the fit, the shorter its duration afterwards, the greater are the grounds for hope that the seizures will eventually cease.

Cases of this last class are to some degree, at any rate, under the child's control. I have several times seen a fit warded off by the threat of the shower bath, or even by calling to the child, and sending it to fetch something in another room. Such cases may indeed pass into ordinary epilepsy, but often, under judicious management, moral rather than medical, they cease, so that one can venture on taking a more hopeful view of them than of others.

And this brings me to the question of what can be done, or rather what can parents do to promote recovery from epilepsy. First of all, do not listen to what you may hear about this medicine or the other being a specific for it. There is no specific whatever for epilepsy, but there are certain remedies which in skilful hands do have a real though limited power to control the frequency and lessen the severity of the attacks. Next, there are cases in which the attacks depend on some definite cause; it may be indigestion, or constipation, or the cutting of the second set of teeth, and on the irritation produced by those teeth being too crowded. Thus, I remember a boy twelve years old, in whom two severe epileptic fits occurred apparently without cause. He was cutting his back grinding teeth, and in the lower jaw the teeth seemed overcrowded. I had a tooth extracted on either side, the fits ceased, and when I last heard of him many years afterwards they had not returned.

Epilepsy often lasts for many years, and no one's memory is retentive enough to be trusted with all the details between the different attacks, the causes which seemed to produce them, the measures which appeared at different times to be of service. I am therefore accustomed to advise people, any of whose children have the misfortune to be epileptic, to write as brief an account as possible of the child's previous history, and to supplement it by a daily record kept in parallel columns of date, food, state of bowels, sleep, medicine, attacks, specifying their character and duration; and general remarks, which would bear on the child's temper and general condition, and in which column any probable exciting cause of an attack would be recorded. It is surprising how much important information is gathered in a few months from such a record kept faithfully.

The diet should be mild, nutritious, but as a general rule unstimulating; and should include meat comparatively seldom, and in small quantities. Some fifty years ago, a very distinguished American physician, Dr. Jackson of Boston, in the United States, insisted very strongly on the importance of a diet exclusively of milk and vegetables in greatly lessening the frequency and severity of epileptic attacks. I believe in the great majority of cases of epilepsy in childhood Dr. Jackson's advice is worth following. And I may add that, while I have little faith in the influence of mere drugs, I have a yearly increasing confidence in that of judicious management, mental and moral, as well as physical.

The first requisite in all cases is a firm and gentle rule of love on the part of those who have charge of the child. As violent and sudden excitement of any kind will often bring on an epileptic seizure, so the influence of the opposite condition in warding off its attacks is very remarkable; and on several occasions I have received patients into the Children's Hospital who were reported to have epileptic seizures several times in a day, and who nevertheless remained a fortnight or more in the institution without any attack coming on. The disorder, however, was not cured, but only kept in check by the gentle rule to which the little ones were subjected. The order goes for much in these cases; the novelty goes for something too, for almost invariably I have found that after a time the apparent improvement becomes less marked, and though they continued better than when they first came to the hospital, the children were still epileptic; the advance of the disease had been retarded, but its progress had not been arrested. The quiet then which suits the epileptic, is not the quiet of listless, apathetic idleness, but the judicious alternation of tranquil occupation and amusement. The mind must not be left to slumber from the apprehension of work bringing on a fit, but the work must, as far as possible, be such as to interest the child. In the occupations of epileptics therefore, pursuits which not merely employ the mental faculties, but also give work to the hands, such as gardening, carpentering, or the tending of animals, are specially to be recommended; and if by these the mind can be kept awake, the grand object of teaching is answered, and backwardness in reading, writing, or those kinds of knowledge which other children at the same age have acquired, is of very little moment. Many epileptics have an indistinct articulation, and almost all have a slouching gait, and an awkward manner. The former can often be corrected to a considerable degree by teaching the child simple chants, which are almost always easily acquired, and practised with pleasure. The latter may be rectified by drilling, not carried out into tedious minuti? but limited to simple movements; and the irksomeness of drill is almost completely done away with by music, while I believe that the accustoming a child to the strict control and regulation of all its voluntary movements is of very great importance indeed as a curative agent.

It is difficult to carry out these minute precautions on which so much depends in the home with other children of the same family. It is therefore, I believe, better for the child, painful though it is to the parents, that he should be placed under the care of some competent person who will devote the whole of his time to the care of the patient.

=St. Vitus's Dance.=--A state of unconsciousness, accompanied with more or less violent involuntary movements, is characteristic of epilepsy. Involuntary movements without loss of consciousness constitute the disorder commonly known as St. Vitus's Dance. It is rare in early childhood, becomes more common after the age of five, and attains its greatest frequency between the ages of ten and fifteen, girls, owing to their more impressionable nervous system, being affected by it more than twice as often as boys.

It seldom comes on in a child previously in perfect health, and strangely enough it occurs with special frequency in children who have before suffered from rheumatism. Sudden shock or fright is often said to have been its exciting cause; but even then the symptoms seldom come at once, but are gradually developed in the course of two or three days. At first, it is noticed that the child has certain odd fidgety movements, usually of one arm, next of the leg of the same side, so that it stumbles in walking, and then the muscles of the face become affected, the child grimacing strangely, and next the limbs of the opposite side become involved, and as things go on from bad to worse, the child becomes unable to hold anything in its hand, to walk, or even to stand, and even if on the ground still writhes about with the strangest contortions of its body. If matters grow still worse, the child becomes unable to put out its tongue, it swallows with difficulty, it loses not only the power of distinct articulation but even the faculty of speech, while the mind itself becomes weakened, the child seems half idiotic, and even though the movements lessen in violence, power over the limbs is lost for the time, and they seem almost paralysed. Happily cases so severe are very rare, and it is rarer still for them to have a fatal termination. Almost invariably recovery takes place by degrees, the movements lessen, swallowing is performed with less difficulty, the power of speech, returns, and the intellect regains its brightness: but the child is left with a special liability to return of the affection, though the first attack is usually the most severe.

Even at the best, however, the disorder is always tedious, as is shown by the fact that its average duration is seventy days. It is very natural, therefore, that parents should be anxious when they see that their child has some awkward or ungainly habit, some odd trick or gesture never noticed before, lest it should be the beginning of this tedious ailment. Now it is well to remember that St. Vitus's dance does not begin with twitching of the muscles of the face, but that its earliest symptoms are involuntary movements of the arms and twitching of the fingers, and that contortions of the face do not come on till afterwards. Movements of this sort too, even when not limited to the face, vary in the course of a few days in the parts which they affect, and show themselves, now in winking the eyes, then in grimacing, in twitching of the muscles of the face or neck, or in some awkward gait or manner. These are all best left unnoticed, for they are almost invariably made worse if the child's attention is called to them. They are, or at least before the days of Board Schools they were, scarcely ever met with among the children of the poor, for they almost invariably depend on mental strain; not of necessity on undue length of the hours of study, or on the difficulty of the tasks imposed, but often on a child's anxiety to make progress and to keep up with his schoolfellows. In corroboration of this being their cause I may say that, contrary to the rule which obtains with St. Vitus's dance, these movements are more frequent in boys than in girls, for the over-mental strain of boys comes earlier; that of girls seldom occurs before the time of transition to womanhood, and its results are then different, though much graver. In cases of this kind, lessening the mental strain is almost always followed by a cessation of the movements; change of air, country amusements, and a generally tonic treatment perfect the cure, and dancing and gymnastics overcome the remains of any awkward habit.

The movements in real St. Vitus's dance do not shift about as these do from one part to another, but tend to involve various parts in succession, without previously ceasing where they had begun.

The relative share which the parents and the doctor take in the treatment of these cases depends to a great extent on their severity. While attention to the state of the bowels, and a generally tonic treatment are almost always needed, gymnastics and drill are often of very great service in the slighter cases; and a very distinguished Paris physician was accustomed to send children thus affected to march round the Place Vend 彪 e, keeping step while the band was playing. The utility of gymnastics turns very much on the degree in which the child is able by attention to control his movements, and when either as in young children fixed attention cannot be roused, or as in severe cases the effort only adds to the child's nervousness, and in consequence increases the movements, they must be given up. All drill and gymnastics are best carried out in class with other children, and regulated not simply by word of mouth, but by a tune or chant. When recovery is in progress gymnastics will then in almost all instances find their place.

Even when drill and gymnastics cannot be practised, regulated movements of the limbs carried out twice a day for ten minutes at a time are of very real service. Another's will here takes the place of that of the patient, and the limbs are thus taught, though far more imperfectly, to act in concert.

Two or three more cautions may still be of service. Do not keep a child out of bed, and force it to try to exert itself when the movements are very severe; continued movement, voluntary or involuntary, fatigues. Let the child lie in bed; it rests there, and the movements, which always cease during sleep, become at once greatly lessened. So important indeed is it to avoid the exhaustion caused by incessant violent movement, that in bad cases it is sometimes necessary to swathe the limbs in flannel bandages, and so to confine them to splints in order to restrain them. Next, do not become over-anxious because the child grows stupid and ceases to talk; intelligence and the power of speech will certainly come back again. And, lastly, do not be impatient and think your medical adviser incompetent because the disorder lasts so long. An average duration of seventy days implies that while sometimes it ceases sooner, in others it lasts much longer than the two weary months of watching and waiting with which in any case you must lay your account.

=Paralysis, or Palsy.=--When speaking of St. Vitus's dance I said that there was a partial loss of power in the limbs as well as an inability to control their movements. After a fit of convulsions, or an epileptic seizure, power over some limb is often lost for a time which may vary from a few minutes to some hours. In the course of some serious diseases of the brain, one of the manifestations of the mischief is the impairment or the loss of power over one arm or leg, rarely over both; and lastly, that terrible disease diphtheria is often followed by a paralysis so general that the patient is sometimes for days unable to move even a finger, although the condition may eventually pass away.

There is, however, a very real paralysis which occurs sometimes in infants and young children. It comes on for the most part quite suddenly, often unaccompanied by any sign of brain disorder, but tending nevertheless to issue in great permanent impairment of the power over the affected limb or limbs, and eventually to interfere with their growth and thus to produce serious deformity.

It is in general impossible to assign any distinct exciting cause for the affection, though the fact that in two-thirds of the cases it occurs between the ages of six months and three years, proves it to be in some way intimately associated with teething. The oldest child in whom I have ever seen it was aged between seven and eight years, and the youngest a little under six months. It is of excessive rarity for the arm alone to be affected, but it is by no means unusual for the legs alone to be paralysed; though in the majority of instances power is lost on one side only, the leg and arm being both involved.

A child goes to bed quite well, or at the worst having seemed slightly ailing and feverish for a day or two, and on waking in the morning it is suddenly discovered that power is lost over one leg or both, or over both arm and leg of one side. The loss of power is at first seldom complete, though neither arm nor leg can be used to any good purpose, and during the ensuing twenty-four hours the palsy often grows worse, and sometimes affects one or both limbs of the opposite side. After that time recovery in general begins. It is now and then speedy, so that in three or four days all trace of the paralysis may have disappeared. This, however, is a fortunate exception to the general rule, which is that amendment is very tardy, showing itself first in the arm, afterwards in the leg, and, if both sides have been affected, more on one side than on the other. Unless the improvement is very rapid, it is almost always only partial, and the palsied limb, though it does not lose sensation, regains but little power; it grows much more slowly than the other, is always colder and wastes considerably, while, some muscles still retaining more power than others, it becomes twisted out of shape, and requires all the skill of the orthop鑞ic surgeon to remedy or at least to lessen the consequent deformity.

It has been ascertained that this form of palsy depends on a state of congestion, or overfilling of the minute blood-vessels of the spinal marrow. When the child gets well the congestion has passed away; but it does this speedily, and recovery is then rapid as well as complete. If it does not soon pass away, other changes take place in the spinal marrow, and recovery is then slow, incomplete, or even does not take place at all.

Remedies are unfortunately of little avail here, but it is evident that when the palsy is quite recent all movement of the limb must be mischievous, and that the congestion of the spinal marrow to which it is due will be most likely to abate under the influence of perfect quiet, rest in bed, and soothing or fever medicines, or of such as are calculated to overcome constipation, or to correct any fault of digestion, while the importance of teething, and the possible expediency of lancing the gums must not be forgotten.

Afterwards comes the time for exercise of the paralysed limb, for friction, for shampooing, for galvanism; all continued perhaps for months or years with unwearied patience, and I must add with reasonable expectations as to the result. The only additional remark which I have to make is this, that to gain any real good from galvanism, a battery must be procured under the direction of some medical man specially skilled in the use of electricity, and the mode of employing it must be learned thoroughly from him. It is merely idle to purchase a toy machine, and, giving it to the nurse to turn the handle for ten minutes twice a day, to fancy that you are making a serious trial of the effects of galvanism. As a mere money question, a costly machine, and several fees paid in order to be thoroughly instructed in the way to use it, is much cheaper than a cripple child.

A few words may not be out of place with reference to cases in which paralysis is mistakenly supposed to exist. Much anxiety is sometimes expressed by parents concerning children who have long passed the usual age without making any attempt to walk; or who having once walked seem to have lost that power. Now it often happens that after any weakening illness a child ceases for some weeks to walk, just as it ceases to talk. The power in both cases was newly acquired, it called for effort which, when strength is regained, will be put forth once more. The same applies to other instances in which children are late in learning to walk; or who, having once walked, leave off walking when a back tooth, or when one of the eye teeth is coming near the surface of the gum, and regaining the power lose it again, or lose at least the desire to exert it more than once during the active progress of teething. But, holding the child under its arms, you have but to put its feet to the ground, and at once it will draw up its legs though it will make no other movement; or take it on your lap and tickle the soles of its feet, and laughing or crying, as the mood takes it, it will move its legs about as freely as you could wish and show that the power is still there, though for the present the child will not take the trouble to exert it.

Gradual loss of power over one or other leg, especially if attended with pain either in the back or in the knee or hip, should always call for attention, and induce you to seek at once for medical advice. Such cases generally occur later in childhood than the conditions of which I spoke in the former paragraph, and may depend on disease of the spine or of the hip-joint, two serious conditions which it needs the medical expert to discover and to treat.

=Neuralgia and Headache.=---In the grown person neuralgia, as many of us know to our cost, is by no means infrequent; in the child it is very rare, and when a child complains of severe pain in the head, or of severe pain to the knee or hip apart from rheumatism, it is almost invariably the sign of disease of the brain in the one case, of the hip-joint in the other. To this rule there are indeed exceptions, but it will always be well to leave it to the doctor to determine--no easy matter by the bye--whether any given case is one of the rare exceptions or not.

There is, however, one form of real neuralgic headache which is by no means rare in children after the commencement of the second dentition, and which sometimes goes on into early manhood or womanhood, when it becomes what is commonly known as sick headache. It is essentially an ailment of development, incidental to the time when the brain is first called on for the performance of its higher functions.

It does not by any means always depend on over-study, though I do not remember meeting with it in children who had not yet gone into the school-room; and I have frequently found it dependent on too continuous application, though the number of hours devoted to study in the course of the day may not have been by any means excessive.

The child's brain soon tires, and the arrangement, so convenient to parents of morning lessons and afternoon play, works far less well for it than if the time were more equally divided between the two.

The attacks not infrequently come on on waking in the morning, and rapidly become worse, the pain, which is almost always referred to the forehead, being attended with much intolerance of light and sound, with nausea, and often with actual vomiting. Like the vomiting of sea-sickness, however, previous stomach disorder has no necessary share in its production, and I may add, indeed, that it is often difficult to assign any special exciting cause for the attack. The suffering is more often relieved by warm or tepid than by cold applications, and not infrequently pressure or a tight bandage greatly mitigates it. In no case does the attack last more than twelve hours--usually not more than half that time; it passes off with sleep, and leaves the patient weak and with a degree of tenderness of the head to the touch.

Such attacks may occur every fortnight, ten days, or even oftener, but their very frequent return, instead of increasing apprehension, should diminish anxiety. A first attack, indeed, may seem as though it threatened mischief, till it is seen how speedily and completely it passes off, and when afterwards a second or a third attack comes on with the same severity of onset, the same rapid worsening, and the same quick passing away, you will feel convinced that the symptoms have no grave meaning.

There is a headache of quite a different kind to which I must for a moment refer, that, namely, which depends entirely on imperfect vision, and for which spectacles are the remedy, not physic. The infirmity is not noticed during the first few years of life, but in later childhood, when a tolerably close attention to study has become necessary. Some of the minor degrees of short-sightedness, and want of power of adaptation of the eyes, such as exists in the aged, soon begin to interfere sensibly with the child's comfort, and the strain to which the eyes are subject produces a constant pain over the brow, the cause of which is often unsuspected.[13]

In all cases, therefore, in which a child complains of constant pain over the brow for which there is no obvious cause, it is well to take the opinion of an oculist, who can best ascertain the power of reading at different distances and with each eye separately, and the real cause of symptoms which had occasioned much anxiety is thus often brought to light.

=Night Terrors.=--Before taking leave of the disorders of the nervous system, I must briefly mention the Nightmare, or Night Terrors of children, which often cause a degree of alarm quite out of proportion to their real importance.

It happens sometimes that a child who has gone to bed apparently well, and who has slept soundly for a short time, awakes suddenly with a sharp and piercing cry. The child will be found sitting up in bed, crying out as if in an agony of fear, 'Oh dear! Oh dear! take it away! father! mother!' while terror is depicted on its countenance, and it does not recognise its parents, who, alarmed by the shrieks, have come into its room, but seems wholly occupied by the fearful impression that has roused it from sleep. By degrees consciousness returns; the child now clings to its mother or its nurse, sometimes wants to be taken up and carried about the room, and by degrees, sometimes in ten minutes, sometimes in half-an-hour, it grows quiet and falls asleep; and then usually the rest of the night is passed undisturbed, though sometimes a second or even a third attack may occur before daybreak.

Seizures of this kind may come on in a great variety of circumstances, and may either happen only two or three times, or may continue to recur at intervals for several weeks. The great point, however, to bear in mind is that they depend invariably on some disorder of the stomach or bowels, and are never an evidence of the commencement of real disease of the brain.

FOOTNOTES:

[11] Reports of the Registrar-General, as quoted at p. 30 of my Lectures on Diseases of Children. The actual numbers are 9,350 under five years old, out of a total of 16,258.

[12] Figures deduced from the 44th Report of the Registrar-General.

[13] Before I called attention to this form of headache in the last edition of my lectures, it had already been noticed without my knowledge, by a friend of mine, Dr. Blache, of Paris, in a very valuable essay on the headaches which occur during the period of growth.

CHAPTER VII.

THE DISORDERS AND DISEASES OF THE CHEST.

In speaking of the ailments which occur during the first month after birth, I have already noticed the peculiarities of breathing in early infancy, and the difficulties that sometimes attend the complete filling of the air-cells of the lungs, and the readiness with which when once filled they become emptied of air and collapse.

On this ground it is therefore needless for me again to enter, and I may pass at once to consider those ailments which rise in increasing importance from a simple cold or catarrh to inflammation of the air-tubes or bronchitis, inflammation of the lung substance, as pneumonia, and inflammation of the membrane which lines the chest and covers the lungs, or pleurisy.

=Catarrh.=--A common cold or catarrh is not one of the ailments of very early infancy. The watery eyes, the sneezing, the cough, the slight feverishness and the heavy head are scarcely met with until after the age of three months; nor, indeed, are they often seen till the child is old enough to run about, to go out for a walk, and to encounter in consequence all the variations of temperature and of damp or dryness inseparable from the English climate.

This, however, is not entirely due to the greater exposure of the child to these influences as it grows older, but in part also to the fact that the lining of the air-tubes is less sensitive in early infancy than it afterwards becomes. The young babe if it catches cold gets snuffles, or stoppage of the nostrils, which first become dry, and then pour out an abundant discharge, which sometimes dries and forms crusts, and causes the child to suck with difficulty, and to breathe uncomfortably and with open mouth. In a few days, however, at the worst this discomfort passes away; and the only additional remark I have to make is, that since obstinate snuffles are sometimes a constitutional disease, the doctor's advice should always be sought if they last longer than a week.

It is needless to describe a cold, but it is much more to the purpose to say how its occurrence is to be prevented, and nine times out of ten the observance of two simple rules will suffice for this. First, take care that there is no great difference between the temperature of the day and of the night nursery. The one should never be above 60? nor the other below 50? and the undressing and the bath should always take place in the warmer room. Second, never let the child wear the same shoes or boots in the house as it does out of doors. The change should be as much a matter of routine as the taking off its hat or its bonnet.

The domestic management of a cold is simple enough. The usual error is the overdoing precautions, the keeping the room too hot, or overloading the child with extra garments, or its bed with extra covering, by which it is kept in a state of feverishness, or of needlessly profuse perspiration.

If, for the first two days of a bad cold, the child is kept in bed, the room being at a temperature of 60? with no extra covering on the bed, but a flannel jacket for the child to wear when it sits up in bed to play, a few drops of ipecacuanha wine several times a day, a warm bath, a linseed poultice to the chest, and a little paregoric at night, with a light diet of rice, and arrowroot, and milk, and a roasted apple, and some orange juice; nine times out of ten, or nineteen out of twenty, the cold will pass away with small discomfort to the child and no anxiety to the parents.

Often a child objects to stop all day in its little cot, but move it to its mother's or nurse's big bed; and with a large tray of toys before it, and a little of the tact which love teaches, the day will pass in unclouded content and cheerfulness.

It must of course be borne in mind that measles set in with all the symptoms of a bad cold, followed on the fourth day by the appearance of the eruption; and, moreover, watchfulness must always be alive to detect increase of fever, hurry of breathing, hardness or extreme frequency of cough, the sign of the irritation of the larger air-tubes having extended and become more severe, the evidence that the case from simple catarrh has become one of bronchitis.

=Bronchitis and Pneumonia.=--It is impossible to enable persons who have not received a medical education to distinguish between a case of bronchitis and one of pneumonia. Neither, indeed, is it of much importance that they should do so, for in both the dangers are of a similar kind, and both call equally for the advice of a skilful doctor.

In bronchitis inflammation affects the lining of the air-tubes, travelling from the larger towards the smaller, and in bad cases extending even to their termination in the minute air-cells. The inflammation leads to the pouring out of a secretion, which by degrees becomes thick like matter, or even very tenacious, almost as tough as though it were a thin layer of skin. If this is very extensive, and reaches to the small air-cells, it is evident that air cannot enter, while that elasticity of the lung which I have already spoken of tends to drive out from the cells the small quantity of air they contained, and the child dies suffocated, partly from the difficulty in the entrance of air, partly from the collapse of air-cells from which the air has been slowly expelled.

In pneumonia or inflammation of the lung-substance the process is different. A portion of one or other lung, sometimes of both, becomes overfilled with blood, or congested, and though the air-tubes themselves are not the special seat of the congestion, yet the air-cells are pressed on by the surrounding swollen substance, and the entrance of air into them is impeded. If the mischief goes further the substance becomes solid and impervious to air, and lastly it becomes softened, its structure destroyed, and infiltrated with matter; the affected part becomes really an abscess, though not bounded by the distinct limits which would shut in an abscess of the hand or the foot. Inflammation, and the formation of an abscess anywhere is, as we know, attended by fever and much general illness, and inflammation of the lung is of course attended by fever and general illness in proportion to the importance of the organ affected. To these, too, must be added all the disturbance inseparable from any ailment which gravely interferes with breathing.

In the great majority of instances inflammation of the lung-substance does not go on to the last stage, and recovery is not only possible, but probable, from congestion and solidification of the organ. Pneumonia, too, usually attacks only a portion of one lung, while in bronchitis the air-tubes of both are always involved. Hence of the two, serious bronchitis is more to be dreaded than serious pneumonia.

Bronchitis is always developed out of previous catarrh, though there is a wide difference between the duration of the preliminary stage and the occurrence of serious symptoms in different cases; while it may be laid down as a general rule that the severity and danger of an attack are in proportion to the rapidity of its onset. An attack of pneumonia, or inflammation of the lung-substance sets in, as a rule, more suddenly, with fever, a temperature of 103?to 105? general distress, headache, not unfrequently delirium; the urgency of which symptoms, the hurried breathing and the short, dry, hacking cough, and the tearless eyes are too often misinterpreted, and the state of the chest not examined.

The doctor, of course, skilled in auscultation, will listen to the chest and give to all these symptoms their true signification. The lesson for the parent to bear in mind is never to neglect in a child the symptoms of what may seem to be but a common cold, but to seek for advice the moment the cough shows any disposition to become hard, or the breathing hurried. Next, when any sudden illness sets in with very high temperature and much general ailing, not to let the disorder of the head, or the delirium, make you shut your eyes to the import of the short cough, the dry eyes, the hurried breathing; and lastly, to remember that, grave though the symptoms may be, the tendency in pneumonia is to eventual recovery, and that in early life bronchitis is the graver of the two diseases.

A caution may not be out of place with reference to cases which may occur during the epidemic prevalence of influenza. A child is sometimes struck down by it, just as grown persons are sometimes, with great depression, extreme rapidity of breathing, and very high fever, which, passing off in a couple of days, leave a state of great exhaustion behind. It is well to bear in mind that such symptoms have no such grave meaning when influenza is prevalent as they would have at another time; and the knowledge of this fact may serve in some degree to control your anxiety.

=Pleurisy.=--It is not possible for anyone, without medical experience, to discriminate between pneumonia, or inflammation of the substance of the lung, and pleurisy, or inflammation of its covering. Some degree of the latter, indeed, very often accompanies the former, and this accounts for the pain which interferes with every attempt of the child to draw a deep breath. When pleurisy comes on independent of affection of the lung-substance, it generally sets in suddenly with severe pain in the chest, and a short hacking cough which causes so much pain that the child tries as much as possible to suppress it. After a few hours the severity of the pain usually subsides, but fever, hurried breathing, and cough continue, and the child, though usually it looks heavy and seems drowsy, yet becomes extremely restless at intervals-- cries and struggles as if in pain, and violently resists any attempt to alter its position, since every movement brings on an increase of its sufferings. The posture which it selects varies much; sometimes its breathing seems disturbed in any other position than sitting straight up in bed; at other times it lies on its back, or one side; but whatever be the posture, any alteration of it causes much distress, and is sure to be resisted by the child.

The variations of posture depend on the seat of the inflammation; the pain depends on the two inflamed surfaces of the membrane rubbing against each other, and accordingly is relieved not merely by the abatement of the inflammation, but also when either the two surfaces become, as they often do, adherent to each other, or when fluid is poured out into the cavity of the chest, and thus keeps them asunder.

I dwell on this, because when fluid is poured out, the most distressing symptoms greatly abate, or even disappear, and parents sometimes put off in consequence sending for the doctor, while yet, if unattended to, the fluid may increase to so large a quantity as to press upon the lung, and so interfere with the entrance of air, or it may, if the mischief is not checked, change into matter, and then have to be let out by tapping the chest, for just the same reason as it may be necessary to open an abscess in any other situation.

Whenever, then, symptoms, such as I have described, come on, send at once for medical advice, and do not let some diminution of suffering, or slight general improvement, lead you to delay.

=Croup.=--I endeavoured to explain, a few pages back, the cause of that peculiar sound which is heard in spasmodic croup. The contraction of the opening of the windpipe changes the sound which passes through it, just as the opening or closing the keys of a wind instrument modifies the sound which it gives forth. But the windpipe is not simply a wind instrument, it is a stringed instrument too, and the strings or vocal cords, as they are termed, give forth, as they vibrate, tones now deeper, now more shrill. The action of this delicate apparatus is readily disturbed, if the nerve-supply to it is disordered by irritation in some distant organ, and then the breathing is accompanied by the peculiar sound of spasmodic croup, or in older children this may show itself in a different way, as in the loud, barking cough heard in some cases of constipation, or of disordered digestion; or another illustration of it is furnished by the loud, long breath--the 'hoop,' which gives its name to hooping-cough. But there is one sound that sometimes attends the breathing of children, which more than any other causes, and justly causes, the greatest anxiety to a mother; and that is the sound which is characteristic of croup.

The word croup, which comes from the Lowland Scotch, signifies merely hoarseness in breathing or coughing, and is therefore, strictly speaking, the name of a sign of disease, rather than that of the disease itself. The peculiar sound is heard in two different conditions--the one in which a child having caught cold, instead of the air-tubes alone being affected, the windpipe, and especially its upper part, becomes congested, and the lining membrane swollen. Partly owing to this, partly owing to its nerve-supply being disturbed, the child breathes noisily and hoarsely, and the cough has a peculiar metallic clangor. In the other case there is not merely the congestion of the windpipe, the disturbed nerve-supply, and the swollen state of the membrane; but in connection with the influence of the special poison of diphtheria, a deposit takes place at the back of the throat, whence it extends to the windpipe, and in many instances even far beyond it, blocking up its canal, and mechanically excluding the entrance of air.

To determine at once to which class a case of croup belongs is so far from easy, that I should advise that on the first sound of voice, or cough, or breathing resembling that of croup, medical advice should at once be sought. I dwell on the difference between the two: the first which has been called false croup, or better catarrhal croup, and the second called true croup, or diphtheritic croup, in order to save much needless apprehension to parents, in whose mind the croupy sound is invariably associated with nothing short of that most dangerous disease--diphtheria.

As a general rule catarrhal croup is rarely met with after the age of six. Children in whom it occurs have either seemed quite well, or at most have been a little ailing for a day or two with cold, and cough, and perhaps slight hoarseness. They go to bed and fall asleep as usual, but the cough, which does not wake them, becomes suddenly noisy, ringing, croupy, and the breathing is speedily attended with a long-drawn sound, half-hissing, half-ringing, and the child soon wakes alarmed, and fighting for breath, the skin bathed in perspiration, the face flushed and anxious. The cough, the difficult breathing, and the struggle for air last for an hour or two, or sometimes all night long, though they gradually subside, at any rate towards the approach of morning, when the child falls asleep, and, but for a somewhat hoarse sounding cough, and a look of fatigue, there are but few signs of all that it has endured.

The attack may not return, or it may recur for two or three successive nights, though in general with lessened severity, the child during the daytime seeming to suffer only from a slight cold, or now and then, and so rarely that I have not known it to occur above once or twice in all my experience, it may end in real inflammation of the windpipe; but not in diphtheria.

Attacks of this kind may recur three, four, or more times even in childhood, while diphtheria has no tendency to recur, but like measles or scarlatina seldom appears more than once, though the rule is subject to more numerous exceptions than are found in the case of the eruptive fevers. Still the fact of an attack of this sort returning should of itself lessen apprehension and make the parents look forward to its issue with less anxiety than that with which they regarded its first occurrence.

A fact which shows how large a part is played by disturbance of the nervous system in these cases is the liability of children who have suffered from it to attacks of asthma, often of great severity as they grow older, while very often after the transition from childhood to youth has passed these attacks too lessen in frequency and severity, and often altogether cease.

There are two measures which, while waiting for the doctor's arrival, may at once be taken, and which sometimes remove the symptoms almost as if by magic, while even were the case one of diphtheria they would still be of some service, and could not possibly do any harm. They are the hot bath, and a full dose of ipecacuanha wine. The former should be as hot as it can be borne, 93?or 94? and the child should be kept in it for five minutes, and the latter should be given in a full dose, as a teaspoonful in warm water every quarter of an hour till free vomiting takes place. How much better soever the child may seem after the use of these remedies, it should still be kept for two or three days under careful medical observation.

=Diphtheria.=--In diphtheria croup is only one, though the most frequent, and one of the most serious, of the many dangerous symptoms which attend it. The croupal symptoms hardly ever come on quite suddenly, but are almost always preceded for some days by slight feverishness, languor, and restlessness, in spite of which the child still amuses itself; and if too young to express its sensations, the slight degree of sore-throat it experiences is manifested rather by a disinclination to take food than by any obvious difficulty in swallowing. There is no cough, nor any change of voice when the child is awake, but when asleep--and the sleep is generally uneasy--it often breathes with its mouth open, it snores slightly, or there is a little hoarse sound accompanying the breathing owing to a trivial swelling of the throat; while, if sought for, there will generally be found a very little enlargement, and a very little tenderness of the glands at the corner of the lower jaw. The eyes are sometimes tearful, there may be slight running at the nose, and the child is said to have a bad cold with slight sore-throat--the most remarkable feature of the case being generally that the depression of the patient is out of proportion to the severity of the local ailment. If now the throat is examined-- and examination of the throat should never be omitted in any case where there is the slightest difficulty of swallowing--nothing may at first be seen but a very little swelling, and some redness of one or other tonsil. In a few hours more, white specks like little bits of curd will be seen first on one tonsil, then on the other, and next these specks will have united to form one continuous layer of a sort of yellowish-white membrane over the palate and tonsils. The examination of the throat, often so difficult when children are ill, is attended with almost none, if while they are well they have been taught the little trick of opening their mouths to show their throat, and of allowing the introduction of a spoon to keep down the tongue, a proceeding which though certainly unpleasant they will almost always readily agree to, like Martha Trapbois, in the 'Fortunes of Nigel,' 'for a consideration.' The deposit on the throat may disappear of its own accord, and not be reproduced, and this even though no treatment has been adopted, and in two or three days the child may be pretty well again, though strength is in general regained less rapidly than might have been expected from the comparative mildness of the attack.

In cases so slight it is no easy matter to recognise the features of a highly dangerous disease; still, out of forerunners so trivial as these, croupal symptoms may be developed, and their advances may be most insidious, and unless both parents and doctor have been closely on the watch they may be surprised all at once by the breathing suddenly becoming very laboured, by that and the cough becoming attended by the sounds characteristic of croup, and by the child's life being in extreme jeopardy, or in danger even beyond the hope of recovery.

It is not that here, as in cases of catarrhal croup, the ailment has really come on suddenly, but that the disease has been silently making unsuspected progress. Whenever then a child, after a few days of slight causeless ailing, accompanied with some little discomfort in swallowing, is seen to have white patches at the back of its throat, do not allow yourselves to be lulled even by their disappearance into a feeling of absolute security. Watch the child, and beg the doctor to watch it carefully, until it is perfectly well again, for though the deposit may have disappeared from the back of the throat it may continue to be formed in the windpipe, and in the somewhat depressed state of the nervous system which attends diphtheria it may not excite that irritation which any such cause would produce in a child in perfect health, and consequently not announce its presence until its amount has become so considerable as to offer an almost insurmountable obstacle to the entrance of air. Any, even the slightest, hurry of breathing, a hissing sound when the child draws its breath, hoarseness of voice, or a ringing cough, should quicken your apprehension of danger, and make you seek for immediate help.

It may be as well, however, to mention here, that not every white speck seen at the back of the throat is of necessity due to diphtheria, but that in some cases of ordinary sore-throat white spots may form on the surface of the tonsils. These white spots are due to the collection at their openings of the secretion formed in the minute glands which beset the surface of the tonsils, and which at these seasons is poured out in greater abundance than usual. They are distinct from each other, and do not coalesce into a membrane; the surface beneath is not the uniform red shining surface on which the membrane in diphtheria has formed, but the separate tiny openings from which the white matter has exuded may be distinctly seen if the surface is wiped with a camel's-hair brush. It is, of course, wise in every case to leave to the doctor the decision as to the nature of the deposit, but it may sometimes relieve needless anxiety to know beforehand that there is another cause besides diphtheria to which white spots at the back of the throat may be due.

There are other dangers, indeed, besides those arising from croup, which accompany diphtheria, though those just mentioned are of all the most frequent. There are cases in which death takes place not from the severity of any local ailment, but from the intense depression of the nervous system. There are other instances too, in which the case assumes what is termed a malignant character; profuse discharge taking place from the nostrils, swallowing being from the first exceedingly difficult, membrane being deposited on the lips, behind the ears, or at the edge of the bowel; death taking place in twenty-four or thirty-six hours from the outset of the first serious symptoms, either in convulsions, or from utter exhaustion.

But the very urgency of such cases must of necessity call for the immediate assistance of the doctor; and my business throughout this book is rather with those points which it is important for a mother to notice, and those things which it behoves her to do.

What does diphtheria depend on? is a question more easily asked than answered. The disease is contagious, as scarlatina is contagious, though not to the same degree. I may add, it is not identical with scarlatina, nor does the one disease protect from the other. It would, perhaps, be too much to say that it is dependent on an unsanitary condition of a town, a village, or a house, but there is no doubt but that, as is the case with cholera, scarlet-fever, or typhus, unsanitary conditions favour its spread, and increase its severity.

Being contagious, it is most important to keep cups, glasses, spoons, towels, and bed-linen separate from those of other inmates of the house, and to remove the patient from any room occupied by other children. Great care too is to be observed, if anyone is standing over the child during a fit of coughing, that none of the membrane which it spits up enters the mouth; and, that if the child's breath is caught, the attendant gargle immediately with a teaspoonful of Condy's fluid in a tumbler of water.

In the next place, as the depression of the nervous system in some cases of diphtheria is quite out of proportion to the local disease, and as children who have not seemed very suffering, have yet been known to die suddenly in an unexpected faint, it is of moment that the child remain constantly in bed from the commencement of the attack till complete convalescence. Nor, indeed, in serious cases is even this precaution sufficient; but in such circumstances not only must the child not be taken out of bed for any purpose, but it must even not be suddenly raised in bed, from a recumbent to a sitting posture. I have, on several occasions, known the neglect of these precautions followed immediately by what cannot but be regarded as the needless death of the patient.

During the illness, there is little for the mother to do, except to try to carry out the doctor's directions, and to give the child constantly little bits of ice to suck, which lessen the swelling of the throat, and relieve the pain and inflammation. If the child knows how to gargle, it should be induced to do so constantly, and finding the relief which this affords, will do so very readily. This is not the time, however, when the lesson 'how to gargle' can be learnt. A thoughtful mother teaches it while the child is well, and if the gargle is composed of raspberry vinegar and water, the lesson is learnt without tears. There comes a time, however, if the disease is at all severe, when gargling is no longer possible, for the muscles of the back of the throat lose their power; but now some medicated solution, employed by means of the spray-producer, may most efficiently take its place.

When croupal symptoms have gone on growing worse and worse, and the child is in the agonies of suffocation, the doctor may propose to open the windpipe, in the hope of giving the child another chance of recovery, and even though the operation fail, of at least lessening its sufferings.

The operation is sometimes objected to by the parents, on the ground of the uncertainty of the result, and the torture of the operation to the child. Now the anguish of a child dying of croup is due to two causes; first, the actual mechanical impediment to the entrance of air produced by the deposit in the windpipe, and secondly, to the spasm of the muscles in the upper part of the windpipe which that deposit produces. How large an amount of distress the latter may produce, anyone can judge for himself, to whom it has ever happened to swallow the wrong way, as it is called. The opening made below the seat of the muscles which close the windpipe, leaves them in perfect rest, and does away with all the suffering produced by spasm, while there is always a fair prospect if the operation is not put off too long, of the deposit being limited to the part above the artificial opening, and of the good being permanent.

It is true that we have no certain means of knowing the extent of the deposit beforehand; it is true also that the operation is not in itself a cure of the disease, but at any rate, it is a reprieve which gives time for remedies to take effect, and at the worst, it substitutes a comparatively painless death for one of intolerable anguish. It can, too, be performed under the influence of chloroform, so that the idea that it adds in any way to the child's distress is unfounded. Who that has seen the calm, happy face, and watched the tranquil sleep of the child after the operation, who before was struggling, with distorted features and agonised countenance, to get a breath of air, but would feel as I do, that I would have it done in a child of mine for the sake of a painless death, even though I knew for certain that it would not prolong life even for an hour?

One additional remark I have to make with reference to the loss of power, or palsy of various muscles, which frequently follows diphtheria. Almost always there is some impairment of power in the muscles of the throat on which the deposit had taken place, and there is, in consequence, a little difficulty in swallowing for a few days. If this should get worse, food and especially drink sometimes return by the nose, and next there may be a slight squint, and the sight may become weakened, and an uncertain tottering gait; and sometimes for a week or two the child may be unable even to stand. In bad cases there is with these symptoms a general loss of nervous as well as of muscular power, though the child may still be fairly cheerful, and ready to amuse itself as well as it can. This condition may last for many weeks before it passes quite away, and if under the mistaken impression that the limbs will gain strength by exercise, the child is allowed to sit up and encouraged to exert itself, recovery will be delayed much longer; and dangerous weakness or fatal exhaustion may suddenly come on.

The inference is too obvious for me to need dwell on it, that repose is the great resource, and quiet waiting the true wisdom.

=Hooping-Cough.=--I need not say much about hooping-cough, for there is scarcely a nursery in which, to everyone's great discomfort, it is not known as a familiar and most unwelcome visitant. It varies remarkably in its importance, being sometimes so slight as scarcely to amount to an illness, but in other instances one of the most deadly of diseases. It causes the death of a fourth of all children who die under the age of five, and three out of four of these deaths take place in infants of less than two years old.

It occurs, however, comparatively seldom during the first three or four months of life, probably because very young children are kept more at home than others, and are thus less exposed to catch it. Though hooping-cough is undoubtedly very contagious, it seems to be communicated only by the breath, and there is absolutely no evidence to show that the clothes of a child suffering from hooping-cough can carry the infection as they might were the child suffering from measles, or smallpox, or scarlet-fever; still less that a person who has visited a room where children are suffering from hooping-cough can convey the disease to another house, or to other children.

The disease derives its name, as everyone knows, from the peculiar sound which attends the cough, and which is due, as is the sound of croup, to spasm of the upper part of the windpipe. It is equally characterised by the cough returning in fits or paroxysms, which end in a long-drawn breath, attended by the hoop. An occasional sound like a hoop, in a young child who has a cold, is not so conclusive of a case being one of hooping-cough as is the recurrence of the cough in fits; for until teething is completed, slight and temporary irritation will suffice to produce a passing spasm of the upper part of the windpipe.

An ordinary attack of hooping-cough begins like a common cold, but as the little ailment passes off, the cough still continues, the fits of coughing become more frequent, last longer, grow severer and more suffocative, and end with the loud long breath, the hoop; while sometimes no sooner is one fit over than another follows it almost immediately, and quiet breathing does not return until the child is tired out by its efforts. Nevertheless, the child's health continues fairly good, and little or nothing ails it during the intervals of the cough. For about a fortnight the cough usually goes on to increase; and during this time the night attacks especially become more frequent. It then for a week or ten days continues stationary, and then declines, a diminution in the frequency and severity of the night attacks being in general the first sign of amendment, and at the end of six weeks from the beginning of the attack the child is in general quite convalescent. Even then, however, a trifling cause will reproduce the characteristic cough for a few days, and not seldom for many months afterwards any cold which the child may catch will be attended by a paroxysmal cough undistinguishable save by its milder character and shorter duration from the previous hooping-cough, though I believe incapable of communicating that disease.

In mild hooping-cough there is little or nothing to be done, save to follow the dictates of common sense, and not to neglect them in quest of some imaginary specific--some vaunted medicine which is said to be a certain cure; or such as shutting up the child in a room the atmosphere of which is charged with the vapour of tar, or of carbolic acid, or of sulphur.

It cannot be too strongly impressed on the minds of parents that there is no specific whatever for hooping-cough; no remedy which will cut it short, as quinine cuts short a fit of ague. The domestic treatment of mild hooping-cough is the domestic treatment of a common cold, implying the same precautions as to the equal temperature of the day and night nursery, the little doses of ipecacuanha at night, but as seldom as possible during the day, in order not to interfere with the appetite and digestion, together with special care to insure the regular action of the bowels. It sometimes happens that after a week or two the severer fits of coughing are followed by vomiting; and the child may lose flesh and strength from inability to retain its food. In these circumstances food must be given, little in quantity, at short intervals, and of a kind that need not remain long in the stomach in order to be digested. Good soup, beef-tea, milk, rice milk, or a raw egg beaten up in milk, and biscuit rather than bread, must take the place of the ordinary meals, and be given twice as often.

The different liniments, and the favourite Roche's Embrocation, are of use when the disease is on the decline, and may also be of service if bronchitis should occur to complicate the hooping-cough, but not otherwise.

Change of air when hooping-cough is on the decline is often of great service, and change even from good air to one less good appears to be sometimes of use; but change in the early stages, or when hooping-cough has become really severe, is but adding another to the already existing dangers.

The danger in hooping-cough arises through the medium either of the head or of the lungs, and through each of them with about equal frequency. The head becomes affected in consequence of the often recurring congestion of the brain, produced, as in spasmodic croup, by the constantly returning interruption to the breathing. In these cases the cough is frequent, and so violent that the child becomes livid during each paroxysm, and that instead of ending in a loud hoop it finishes by a fit of convulsions or by the child sinking into a state of semi-insensibility. Increased violence of the cough, with suppression of the hoop, is always a bad omen in hooping-cough.

On the other hand, when the cough becomes complicated with bronchitis, it ceases to recur in distinct fits which leave behind them intervals of comparative, or of absolute ease. The hurried breathing which precedes and follows a fit of coughing never entirely subsides, while each returning cough aggravates the irritation and inflammation of the air-tubes, and the child's condition becomes the very dangerous one of hooping-cough complicated with bronchitis.

So long as a child seems pretty well in the intervals between the fits of coughing, as the hurried breathing subsides after each to a natural frequency, as a long loud hoop follows each cough, as vomiting takes place only after a fit of coughing and never in the intervals, as the child becomes flushed only and not livid during a cough, and recovers itself perfectly afterwards, as it does not complain of constant headache, nor spits blood, nor has nose-bleeding, nor is feverish, nor depressed, nor drowsy, you may feel happy about it. When any of the symptoms just enumerated show themselves you have reason for grave solicitude, and the child requires daily medical watching.

One word in conclusion. A child who has recently had hooping-cough is more liable than another to be attacked by chicken-pox or measles; and, moreover, imperfect recovery from hooping-cough is apt, especially if there is any tendency to consumption in the family, to be followed by consumptive disease.

=Asthma.=--Asthma, attended by distress of breathing quite as considerable as in the grown person, is by no means unusual in the child. Recovery from it is far more likely to take place in the latter, since it is almost always independent of those diseases of the heart or lungs, which in the former occasion or aggravate it. It belongs to the class of what has been termed nervous asthma and is observed with special frequency in children who, when younger, had been liable to catarrhal croup; spasm of the air-tubes having taken the place of the previous spasm of the windpipe. Independently of that antecedent it comes on sometimes about the time of the second teething in nervous and impressionable children, in whom an attack may be produced by indigestion, constipation, or over-fatigue. It is also by no means rare in children in whom that skin affection, eczema, of which I have already spoken, outlasts the time of infancy, and becomes general and severe. The improper performance of the functions of the skin seems to cause a peculiar sensitiveness of the air-tubes, and to render them liable to the occasional occurrence of that spasm which produces asthma. These cases are less hopeful than others, and the liability to the attacks ceases only when the skin-affection has been completely cured; a reason this for not neglecting eczema in infancy and early childhood. Sometimes, too, it follows frequently-recurring attacks of bronchitis, and, though less often than might be expected, it succeeds severe hooping-cough, and in these two conditions the prospects of recovery are less hopeful than in the others.

When asthma occurs in childhood, the first point is to ascertain the cause on which the attack depends; and it is worth any amount of care to discover and remove it; for if what may be called the asthmatic habit is not formed, the attacks will, in the majority of instances, cease between the ages of twelve and fifteen. Bad habits of the body are, however, as difficult to get rid of as bad habits of the mind, and the boy who grows up an asthmatic youth is very unlikely to get rid of the disorder in later life.

It is in that form of asthma which succeeds to frequent attacks of catching cold, and in which bronchitis precedes or accompanies each seizure, that change of climate is most useful. In the majority of instances a moderately sheltered seaside place, with a sandy soil such as Bournemouth, is the best, and a few years' residence there not infrequently overcomes every disposition to asthma through the whole remainder of the patient's life. To this, however, there are exceptions, and I have seen instances in which residence at Bournemouth and in the Riviera have failed, but where a perfect cure has been wrought by the cold, still air of Davos.

=Diseases of the Heart.=---=Malformed Heart.=--Every now and then one sees a little babe, carefully wrapped up in its nurse's arms to shield it, even on a warm day, from the air; and, on removing the shawl which covered it, one is struck by the sight of a little pale pinched face, with a livid ring around the mouth, and a blue instead of a rosy tint of lips and fingertips, as though perished with cold. The babe wakes on being disturbed, and gives a faint short cry of distress; the livid hue of its surface deepens, it struggles feebly, its mouth twitches as though convulsions might be coming on. Soon, however, these symptoms subside, the babe smiles again, is cheerful, and save for the tints of its face and lips, it looks like other infants, but frailer.

This condition has a name in medical writings, from a Greek word expressive of the blue tint which characterises it, and is called cyanosis. It depends on the blood not having undergone completely those changes in the lungs which take place in the healthy state. The blood, as it returns through the veins to the right side of the heart, is of a deep purple hue. The right side of the heart contracting sends it to the lungs, where, in the minute vessels of the air-cells, it is purified, and returns vivified by the oxygen a bright scarlet stream, to be distributed by the arteries over the whole body; and thence to return once more for fresh purification to the right side of the heart. Before birth, the blood does not run the same course, but is purified within the mother's body, the blood running through channels which close with the first breath the infant draws. The previously existing communication between the two sides of the heart ceases at the same time as the new channels are opened, by the shutting of a thin valve which had hitherto allowed the blood to pass from one side to the other.

Sometimes this closure fails to take place, or takes place but imperfectly; sometimes, in addition, the channels which should be disused after birth remain open still; and sometimes also the heart is otherwise imperfectly formed, and a large communication exists between the two sides of the heart, which long before birth ought to have been firmly partitioned off from each other.

According to the freedom of communication between the two sides of the heart, there is more or less ready intermingling of the impure blood with that which is already purified; and this is betokened by the greater or less severity of the symptoms which I have described. When the heart is very malformed, and the blood consequently is very impure, life is but a short agony which ends in a few weeks; some slight movement, some little accidental cold deranging altogether the imperfect machinery, and bringing it to a sudden standstill. Between this and the slightest cases there are all shades of difference, till, in the latter, a smaller power to maintain warmth, a less rapid growth, a smaller muscular development, a feebler power, a hurry of breathing on exertion, or in ascending a hill, or in going up a staircase, are all, except the sounds which the educated ear detects of the blood passing through its devious course, that tell of nature having, in this instance, ill done her handiwork.

The one most natural question to which, in every instance, the doctor has to reply is this: 'Will he or she outgrow it?' To this the answer is, 'Yes,' and 'No.' In the worst cases the answer is obviously no; and in none does yes imply a recovery so complete as to leave no trace behind, and to make the child heartwhole. But short of this, in many instances much may be hoped for. There is, as I shall have occasion again to repeat, a power in the growing heart to adapt itself in large measure to conditions other than those of perfect health. The channels, through which the blood ought not to flow, may shrink though they may not entirely close; the valve may shut more completely than at first the opening between the two sides of the heart; all inconveniences may lessen, and the child may at last become scarcely aware of the difference between himself and others. But for any such result, or for anything approaching it to be attained, certain conditions are absolutely essential which it is seldom easy to induce parents to observe. Whatever can hurry the circulation is most carefully to be avoided. The child must be kept strictly out of the way of hooping-cough, measles, or any other fever; must be shielded from every risk of catching cold, and having smaller power of maintaining its warmth than others have, must be specially warmly clad, and must live in rooms at a temperature of 60 deg. Fahr., all the year round. Great attention must be paid to the state of the bowels, so that constipation may not necessitate violent efforts to relieve them.

Moreover, for years the child must be carried upstairs; when old enough to take part in games, it must not be allowed to join in any which call for violent exertion, such as cricket, or lawn tennis, nor ride any other than a quiet pony at a gentle pace.

It depends entirely on the parents whether, for the sake of a very great but far-off good, they will strictly observe these rules. The difficulty will not arise on the child's part, for it is not hard for those who have had charge of it from babyhood to bring it up to quiet pursuits and quiet amusements, till it seeks no others, and, like the little cage-bred bird, does not care to emulate the flight of others stronger on the wing.

=Inflammation of the Heart.=--The above remarks do not comprise all that is to be said about heart-affection in early life. Inflammation may attack the investing or the lining membrane of the heart at all ages, may produce in the child the same suffering as in the grown person, and may tend to destroy life in a similar manner. The causes, indeed, which produce heart disease, are far more frequent in the grown person than in the child, and advancing age brings with it changes which, wholly apart from active inflammation, produce grave forms of disease unknown in early life. There is, however, one cause of heart disease which is far more frequent in childhood and early youth than in later life, namely, rheumatism. Eight out of ten of all cases of heart disease under the age of fifteen are of rheumatic origin, and in eighteen out of twenty cases of acute rheumatism under that age, whether slight or severe, the heart becomes more or less involved. Now and then, though rarely, the heart becomes affected in the course of scarlatina, and still more seldom in the course of the other fevers, and every now and then affection of the heart is associated with some other form of inflammation of the chest.

Pain is by no means a constant attendant on it, but fever, more or less considerable, a quickened pulse, and hurried breathing are all but invariable, and one great reason for seeking the immediate help of the doctor is, that his skilled ear may at once detect by the altered sounds the heart-affection at its very outset, and employ the measures calculated to arrest its progress.

Death in the acute stage of a first attack of inflammation of the heart is of extreme rarity, but the damaged heart is liable to returns of acute mischief, any one of which may prove fatal. Independently of this, life with diseased heart is one of suffering, attended as it is by symptoms similar in kind, though not identical with those which I have already mentioned as attendant on malformation of the organ.

The hopeful element, however, to which I have already referred as present in cases of malformed heart, exists here in even a greater degree; since repair of injury is possible, while the reconstitution of an organ faulty from birth is obviously beyond nature's power.

I can but repeat the directions already given as to the importance of allowing the heart as much rest, and giving it as little work, as is possible with a never-resting organ; and this with the added motive for perseverance furnished by the happy issue which may be hoped for as its reward.

One word I must add about the occasional occurrence of irregular action of the heart during the years of growth, especially from the age of ten to fourteen. This is often quite independent of any disease, and ceases when with added strength the nervous system becomes less impressionable.

CHAPTER VIII.

DISEASES OF THE ORGANS OF DIGESTION.

=Manner of Performance of Digestion.=--The organs situated in what is called in medical language the abdomen, have in the child no other duty to perform than such as subserve the processes of digestion and nutrition. The saliva secreted by the appropriate glands in the mouth, mixing with the food, facilitates the further changes which take place in the stomach. In the stomach the food is acted on and dissolved by the gastric juice or pepsin, which is poured out by an almost infinity of minute tubes, or follicles as they are termed. When the stomach has done its work, its contents in a semi-fluid state pass into the small intestine, and mix there with the bile, the secretions from the intestines themselves, and with those of the large gland, the pancreas (in culinary language known as the sweetbread), which seems to have the special power of dissolving fatty matters. As the food, thus acted on, travels along the intestines, whose constant movement facilitates the passage of their contents from above downwards, its elements are taken up, partly by the blood-vessels, partly by innumerable small vessels, called absorbents from their power of imbibing fluids, and lacteals, from the milky hue of the fluid within them when first absorbed. The fluid taken up by the blood-vessels is conveyed to the liver; that taken up by the absorbents to the mesenteric glands, and in these organs further changes take place in it, which fit it to be received into the mass of the circulating fluid. With this it is carried to the right side of the heart, and thence to the lungs and, lastly, from them to the left side of the heart, whence it is distributed, the great life and health giver, to the rest of the body. The useless inconvertible material, leaving every available element behind, is got rid of, either in a solid form by the bowels, or in a fluid form by the kidneys; and thus as long as life lasts there goes on more or less perfectly the wonderful process of constant change, of constant renewal, and during childhood and youth, of constant increase of size and stature.

Incomplete as this sketch is, it may yet suggest how readily one part of this complex machinery may be thrown out of gear, and further how not one part can suffer without all being disordered. Solid food given to the child before it has cut its teeth, enters the stomach unreduced to pulp by the grinders, and unmixed with the saliva, which should help its solution, and which the undeveloped salivary glands do not yet furnish. Too large a quantity of food, or food of an unsuitable character, on which the gastric juice cannot act readily, may pass into a state of fermentation; vomiting, flatulence, sour and offensive breath will be the result, and the food will pass into the intestine unprepared to be acted on by the bile. Exposure to cold, or the opposite condition of excessive heat, may disturb the action of the liver, and interfere with the secretion of bile; and the food will then pass along the intestine in a state unsuitable for absorption. Or, again, the mesenteric glands may be irritated by long-continued imperfect performance of the earlier stages of digestion, or their structure may be altered, and mesenteric disease, or consumption of the bowels, as it has been termed, may result. From want of muscular power, or from want of care on their part who have charge of the child, the bowels may become habitually constipated. Health will then suffer, if the child carries about with it for days together matters which can serve no useful purpose, but which are to the body what an ill-kept dustbin is to the rest of the house. Lastly, if the kidneys perform their duties imperfectly in consequence of exposure to cold, or of the changes which some diseases, such as scarlatina, sometimes bring about in their structure, the blood will be imperfectly purified; dropsy and various forms of inflammation may result; or the brain and nervous system may be disordered, and death in convulsions may attest the dangerous nature of this blood-poisoning.

It would take too long to go in detail through all the phases of disordered digestion in early life. Much has been already anticipated in a former part of this book, especially with reference to the troubles of digestion in infancy and early childhood. There is, indeed, but one form of indigestion whose characters are so special as to require that I should enter into any detail with reference to it.

=Dyspepsia of Weakly Children.=--Children from the age of about three to ten years, whose health has been impaired by an attack of typhoid, or, as it is commonly called, infantile remittent fever, or who belong to a weakly family, or to one, some of whose members have shown a disposition to consumptive disease, are sometimes martyrs to indigestion. It does not need with them any special error of diet, or any casual exposure to cold to disorder their digestion; but every two or three weeks, even under the most scrupulous care, they lose their appetite, their tongue becomes thickly coated with yellow fur, their breath offensive, their bowels constipated, the evacuations being either very white or very dark, and frequently lumpy, and coated with a thin layer of mucus from the bowel, which also appears in shreds at the bottom of the utensil. With this condition, too, there is some, though not considerable, feverishness, and the urine becomes turbid on cooling, and throws down a reddish-white deposit, which disappears if heated. At the end of two or three days of rest in bed, of a diet of beef-tea and milk, with no solid food, with simple saline medicines, mild aperients, and perhaps a single small dose of calomel, the symptoms pass off; but return again and again at uncertain intervals, and without any obvious cause.

In these cases, the children almost always, when in their ordinary health, have a peculiar patchy condition of the tongue, one part of it being covered with a thin white coating, through which little red points project, while another part is of a vivid red, and looks raw and shining, as though it had been scalded, while the red points, or the papill? as they are termed, project above its surface like so many pins' heads. Children in whom this condition exists, require much watching and much care. I have dwelt upon it in order to impress on parents the conviction that it is not a state to be cured, once for all, even by the most skilful doctor, but that years are needed to eradicate a bad habit of the body, as much as to cure a bad habit of the mind.

=Jaundice.=--I have already spoken of the jaundice of new-born infants; but a sluggish condition of the liver, accompanied by very white or pale evacuations, constipation, and loss of appetite, with a sallow tint of the skin, and sometimes even with actual jaundice, are by no means uncommon during the first ten years of childhood. Neither condition is serious; that of actual jaundice occurs mostly in the summer, and is then connected with the sudden onset of hot weather. When severe, it may be associated with some degree of feverishness, with dizziness, and complaint of headache, and occasionally with vomiting, while the child rests ill at night, or awakes in a state of alarm, and these symptoms sometimes give rise to the fear that the child is about to be attacked by water on the brain. But the following consideration may serve to calm anxiety on that score. The attack is not preceded, as water on the brain is almost invariably, by several days or even weeks of failing health. It is not attended by heat of head, nor by intolerance of light, nor by constant nausea; and the belly is full rather than shrunken. When to these symptoms are added tenderness on the right side, high-coloured urine and white evacuations, you may set your mind at rest, even before the yellow colour of the skin, which appears in a day or two, stamps the case unmistakably as one of jaundice.

My business is, as I have said more than once, the endeavour to describe the symptoms of disease, to explain their nature, to indicate the principles to be observed in attempting their cure, and not to lay down definite rules for their treatment, with the idle expectation that I could thus enable every mother to be her children's doctor.

=Diarrh[oe]a.=--I have, therefore, comparatively little to say about diarrh[oe]a in children, important though it is, for its symptoms force themselves on the notice even of the least observant. There are, however, a few points concerning it worth bearing in mind. Before the commencement of teething, diarrh[oe]a is almost always the result of premature weaning, or of a diet in some respect or other unsuitable. As soon as teething begins, the liability to diarrh[oe]a increases greatly, and cases of it are more than twice as frequent, and twice as fatal, between the ages of six and eighteen months as they were in the first six months of life; while, as soon as teething is over, their number immediately declines again to the half of what it was during the continuance of that process. The practical conclusions to be drawn from these facts are that looseness of the bowels during teething is not a desirable occurrence to be promoted, as some mistakenly imagine, but a risk to be by all means avoided, and I may add, when it does take place, far less easy to control than constipation is to remedy. And next, that in order to prevent its occurrence, care should be taken to make changes in the diet of a child, not during the time when a fresh eruption of teeth is taking place, but during one of the pauses in that process. There are certain seasons of the year when diarrh[oe]a is specially prevalent, independent of any change in diet, or alteration, in any respect, of the circumstances in which the child is placed. Thus, in May, June, and July, diarrh[oe]a is twice as prevalent among children at all ages as in November, December, and January; and in August, September, and October, its prevalence is three times as great as during the winter months. The high mortality of children in the summer months is due almost entirely to diarrh[oe]a, and even the bitter Northern winter of a city like Berlin is a third less fatal to infants and young children than the heat of its short summer.

The next point to remember is that mere looseness of the bowels is never to be regarded during the first three years of life as of no importance; for I have seen infants die exhausted from its continuance, even though the examination of the body after death showed almost no sign of disease. Doctors distinguish two forms of diarrh[oe]a: the simple, or, as it is technically called, catarrhal diarrh[oe]a; and inflammatory diarrh[oe]a, or dysentery. The one may pass into the other, just as a common cold, or catarrh, may pass, if unattended to, into a dangerous bronchitis.

Simple diarrh[oe]a usually comes on gradually, and is some days before it grows severe, or passes into the more dangerous dysentery. Simple precautions will often arrest its progress, and, among them, rest in bed is one of the most important. Over and over again I have known a diarrh[oe]a which had continued in spite of all sorts of medicines so long as the child was running about, cease at once when the child was kept for a couple of days in bed. The reason of this is obvious; constant movement of the intestines themselves, which serves so important a part in maintaining due action of the bowels, is increased by the upright position and by movement, and is reduced to a minimum by the horizontal position. A second precaution concerns the diet; solid food and animal broths should for a time be discontinued, and arrowroot, milk and water, and rice substituted for it, for a day or two, with isinglass jelly, and the white decoction of which I have already spoken. It is not always that astringents are suitable at the beginning of an attack, and the sending to the neighbouring chemist for diarrh[oe]a medicine, which often contains an unknown quantity of opium, is always risky, frequently mischievous. In a first attack of diarrh[oe]a, the doctor should always be consulted, for when it is associated with disorder of the liver a mercurial may in the first instance be needed, or possibly very small doses of a saline medicine, such as Epsom salts, with the addition of a few drops of the tincture of rhubarb; or, again, if the diarrh[oe]a sets in with profuse watery discharges, sulphuric acid for the first few hours is often of extreme service. It is at a later time that direct astringents commonly have their use; and the mother, who in her child's first attack of diarrh[oe]a has had the advice of a judicious doctor, will often be helped by him to manage for herself slight returns of the ailment.

Inflammatory diarrh[oe]a, or dysentery, not only follows the continuance of the simpler forms of the disease, but sometimes in the hot months of summer or autumn sets in suddenly with violence. It then frequently commences with vomiting, and the stomach may continue so irritable for twenty-four hours as not to retain even a teaspoonful of cold water. At the same time the over-action of the bowels sets in, and twenty or thirty evacuations may be passed in twenty-four hours. The motions soon lose their natural character, and become watery, slimy, and mixed with blood. They are at first expelled with violence, afterwards with much pain, effort, and often fruitless straining. With these local symptoms, the child, as might be expected, is very ill, feverish, and stupid, though without sound sleep, much exhausted, and its nervous system so disturbed as to occasion frequent twitchings of the fingers and of the corners of the mouth, while sometimes actual convulsions take place. The thirst is intense, the child calling constantly for cold water, and crying out for more the moment the cup is taken away from its lips; while the loss of flesh and the exhaustion are more rapid than in any other disease with which I am acquainted. The fat happy babe of four and twenty hours before is scarcely to be recognised in the miserable little being, with sunken lustreless eyes, and wizened features, and miserable countenance, lying in a state of half-stupor, sensible only to pain, which yet rouses it but to utter a moan, and then sinks again into silent suffering. I can well believe what we are told, that in some countries this, the so-called Summer Complaint of many of the American cities, sometimes carries off children in a few hours.

If a fatal termination does not take place speedily, the disease passes into the chronic stage, the diarrh[oe]a diminishing in frequency, but the pain and straining, and the unhealthy character of the evacuations persisting. Ulceration of the bowels has taken place, emaciation becomes extreme, and the child often sinks at the end of several weeks, worn out by suffering; while recovery, doubtful at the best, is always very slow. But I need not pursue this subject further: enough has already been said to show how little infantile diarrh[oe]a is a disorder for domestic management.

=Peritonitis=, or inflammation of the membrane covering the bowels and lining the cavity of the belly, is of excessive rarity in its acute form; and is attended by such general illness and such severe local suffering, that it is impossible to overlook it or to misapprehend its gravity. Severe pain in the belly is sometimes complained of by children, and is due to what is termed colic, a spasm of the bowels which is generally associated with constipation. The great test of the cause of the pain is furnished by the presence or absence of tenderness on pressure. The pain of colic is relieved by gentle pressure and gentle rubbing. The pain of inflammation in any degree and of any kind is aggravated by them. This applies also to cases, not indeed very common, in which inflammation is set up by some small body, such as a cherry-stone getting fixed in a little offshoot or appendage of about the size and length of the little finger, connected with the commencement of the large bowel, and producing ulceration. In these circumstances the bowels are confined, there are nausea and sickness, together with pain and tenderness of the belly, especially on the right side. The disease is a very dangerous one, and often proves fatal in the course of a few days. I refer to it because I have often seen it overlooked both by parents and doctors at its outset, since the pain then is often not severe nor the tenderness intense, and because I have seen the patient's condition rendered hopeless by strong aperients being given to overcome the constipation which was supposed to be all that ailed the child. I repeat then the caution, never to overlook the existence of tenderness, never to attempt to treat a case in which it is present; but always to call in medical advice, and above all always to abstain, unless ordered by a medical man, in every such case from the use of aperients.

=Large Abdomen.=--I must not leave the subject of disorder of the digestive organs without some reference to a condition which often excites much needless anxiety among mothers, namely, the large size of a child's belly. This is sometimes supposed to be a certain evidence of the presence of worms, at other times to be a positive proof of the existence of grave disease, especially of disease of the mesenteric glands, or glands of the bowels as they are popularly termed. It is evidence of neither the one nor the other.

If you go into a gallery of the old masters, and look at any of the pictures of angels which are generally to be seen there in such abundance, you will probably be struck in the case of all the child angels by what will seem to you the undue size of their abdomen. You will notice this even in the works of painters who, like Raphael, most idealise their subjects, while in those of others who, like Rubens, interpret nature more literally, the apparent disproportion becomes grotesque; or, in the coarser hands of Jordaens, even repulsive.

These painters were, after all, true interpreters of nature. In infancy and early childhood the abdomen is much larger comparatively than in the grown person. For this there is a twofold cause; the larger size of the liver on the one hand, and the smaller development of the hips on the other. In a weakly child this appearance is exaggerated by its want of muscular power, which allows the intestines to become much distended with air. If the child is not merely weakly but also ricketty, the contracted chest will leave less room than natural for the lungs, while at the same time the ordinary development of the hips being arrested by the rickets, the disproportion is further increased both by that and by the flatulence due to the imperfect digestion with which the condition is almost always associated.

In no case need the mere size of the abdomen occasion grave anxiety, so long as when the child lies upon its back the abdomen is uniformly soft, nor so long as even if tense it is not tender, and as it everywhere gives out a hollow sound like a drum when tapped with the finger.

It is not for a moment meant that no notice is to be taken, nor opinion asked, as to the cause of excessive size of the abdomen, for its distension may be due to real disease; but it is yet worth while to remember that its mere size is not of itself evidence of disease, nor cause of grave anxiety.

=Worms.=---There is no mistaking or overlooking the existence of worms when they are really present. Their presence, however, is often suspected without any sufficient reason. Ravenous or uncertain appetite, indigestion, flatulence, undue size of the abdomen, a dark circle round the eyes, itching of the nose and of the entrance of the bowel, a coated tongue, and offensive breath are no real proof of the presence of worms, and do not justify the frequent repetition of violent purgatives or of so-called worm medicines. The only real proof of the presence of worms is their being seen in the evacuations.

The worms commonly found in children are either the round-worm, which resembles the earth-worm, the thread-worm, or the tape-worm; the appearance of each of which is clearly indicated by its name. None of them are spontaneously generated in the body, but they are all introduced from without; their eggs, or, as they are technically called, their ova, being swallowed unperceived in some article of food, or drink. A proof of this is afforded by the fact that an infant, so long as it is nourished exclusively at the breast, never has worms.

The round-worm occasions the fewest symptoms, and is rather an object of disgust than of grave importance, at least in this country, where it seldom happens that more than two or three are present. In other countries, as some parts of Italy, for instance, where the drinking water is bad and stagnant, they are sometimes found in great numbers, as thirty or forty, and it is then not easy to determine whether the symptoms which accompany them are produced by the worms, or by the unwholesome character of the water in other respects.

They appear to live on the contents of the intestines, and do not adhere to them, as the tape-worm does, and hence their comparative harmlessness, and they have no power, as has sometimes been mistakenly imagined, of perforating the bowels, and of thus producing grave mischief.

The thread-worm is the commonest variety of these creatures, and has the peculiarity of inhabiting the lowest twelve inches of the bowel, where it produces much irritation and causes very distressing itching. It is often present in great numbers, and is so rapidly reproduced, that in a week or two after it has been apparently got rid of, it may again be found as numerous as before. Certain articles of food seem to favour its development, such as pastry, sugar, sweets, beer, fruit, and anything which is apt to undergo fermentation, and thereby to impart to the evacuations a specially acid character. These worms are often accompanied with more or less marked symptoms of indigestion, but otherwise the local irritation is usually the only indication of their presence. They produce, indeed, such disturbance of the nervous system as may attend indigestion in any of its forms, but I have never but once known convulsions occur apparently due to their presence in great numbers, and ceasing on their expulsion; and this was in a child between eighteen months and two years old.

The tape-worm is developed in the human body from a minute germ or ovum; one form of which exists in the flesh of the bullock, the other in that of the pig; and which seems to require for its growth the favouring conditions of warmth and moisture which are found in the intestines. It fixes itself to the lining of the bowels by means of its mouth, which is furnished with minute tentacles, and it thus derives its support from the juices which it imbibes. The head is so small as not to be seen distinctly without a magnifying glass; and immediately beyond it the jointed body begins; at first, scarcely bigger than a thread of worsted, but gradually enlarging, till at the distance of three inches it is an eighth of an inch wide, and thence rapidly widens till each joint is half an inch wide, and from a third to half an inch apart. It does not exceed these dimensions, even though it may grow to the length of four or six yards. Portions of it, sometimes a yard or two in length, are thrown off from its lower end occasionally, and this occurrence often gives the first indication of its presence, the worm continuing to grow as before, and fresh portions being detached from time to time. It does not appear that the worm has the power of reproducing itself; hence its French name of ver solitaire, and the occasional presence of two or three would seem to be due to the development of two or three distinct ova within the intestine.

Deriving as it does its support from the system of the child, and not as the other worms do from the contents of the bowel, the tape-worm often produces graver inconveniences. It sometimes causes uncomfortable colicky sensations, which may even be very distressing, and the disorders of digestion which accompany it are often very considerable; certainly more so than in the case of the other varieties of worms; but I have seen no instance of convulsions which could be attributed to them, notwithstanding the generally received opinion to the contrary.

When the existence of worms is suspected, one or two doses of a simple aperient, such as castor oil, repeated two days successively, seldom fail to produce evidence of their presence; which in the case of tape-worm is also furnished by the spontaneous detachment of some of the joints. It must be remembered, however, that until the head has been detached from its connection with the bowel, nothing has been gained, and the tape-worm will in a short time grow again. To obtain the detachment of the head it is necessary that any worm medicine should be given when the intestines are empty. I am, therefore, always accustomed to give a dose of castor oil about two hours after the child's mid-day meal; and to send the child to bed as soon as the aperient begins to act, and to give it no more food except a biscuit and a little milk and water during the rest of the day. In the early morning, the special worm medicine is given, and over and over again I have known the worm to be brought away completely after many previous failures. When the smallness of the joints shows that the greater part of the worm has been thrown off, and that little more than the head remains, it is necessary to have recourse to the unpleasant proceeding of mixing the evacuations with water, and then straining them through muslin, in order that the doctor may by means of the microscope make out whether or no the head has been really detached. This is no question of mere curiosity, but a matter of the gravest moment, since nothing has been really gained so long as the head of the worm remains adherent to the bowel.

Precautions such as these are not needed in the case of the other kinds of worms. Thread-worms, however, are best attacked in their habitation; that is to say, in the lower bowel, by means of lavements. It is, therefore, desirable before they are administered that the bowels should be emptied by a dose of castor oil.

The only other caution which remains for me to give refers to the peculiar effect which salicine, a very valuable medicine, especially in the case of thread-worms, has upon the urine. It sometimes turns the urine of a greenish-yellow, often of a red colour, as though it were mixed with blood. The appearance, however, has no grave meaning, but is due simply to a chemical action of the medicine on the colouring matter and salts of the urine.

There still remain some local ailments of parts connected with the process of digestion, concerning which a few words must be said.

=Ulcerated Mouth.=---First, with reference to the sore-mouth of children. I have already noticed a form of inflammation and ulceration of the gums sometimes met with during teething, but the sore-mouth of which I am now about to speak is often quite independent of that process; though it may sometimes be found associated with it, and is indeed rarely met with after five years of age. In almost all instances it is preceded and attended with symptoms of indigestion, during the course of which the mouth becomes inflamed, hot and red, and small very painful shallow ulcers with sharp-cut edges, and a little yellowish deposit on their surface, appear at the edge of the tongue, on the inside of the mouth, and especially on the inside of the lower lip, and the adjacent surface of the gum. Successive crops of these little ulcerations not unfrequently appear, so that for many weeks the child may be kept by them in a state of extreme discomfort; swallowing, and even speaking being the occasions of considerable suffering.

It is seldom that nursery remedies, and the so-called cooling medicines, though often of some service, suffice to get rid of the ailment, which for the most part needs judicious medical treatment, and local as well as constitutional measures. Now and then this condition comes on in the course of measles, and is then sometimes of serious importance.

In the other form, the disease is usually limited to the gums, and affects especially those of the front of the lower jaw, which become swollen, ulcerated at their edges, where a very ill-smelling deposit takes place of a dirty white or greyish colour, the surface beneath being spongy, swollen, raw, and bleeding. The ulceration sometimes extends so as to lay bare a large part of the sockets of the teeth; but though loosened they seldom drop out. Coupled with this, the glands at the angle of the jaw are swollen, and the child dribbles constantly a large quantity of horribly offensive saliva. In the children of the well-to-do classes the condition is seldom seen except in a slight degree; but even when severe it is rarely accompanied by any grave disorder of the general health. It seems to tend, whether treated or left to itself, slowly to get well; but its progress to a natural cure is extremely tedious, and the gums are left by it for a long time spongy, bleeding easily, and only very imperfectly covering the teeth.

Anxiety is sometimes excited by this condition; it being supposed that the white deposit on the edge of the gum implies some relation between it and diphtheria. This is not so, for though this peculiar ulceration of the gums has now and then been found associated with diphtheria, the nature of the two diseases is essentially different. It is, however, always wise to call in medical advice in order to settle this important question, and the more so, since there is one remedy, the chlorate of potass, which, in appropriate doses, acts upon the condition almost as a charm.

I say nothing about a dreadful form of inflammation of the mouth which ends in mortification, because it is of infinite rarity except among the destitute poor, and even among them it is very seldom seen except as a consequence of measles, or of some kind of fever. It is only among the very poor that I have seen it, and even among them it has come under my notice only ten times in the whole course of my life.

There is a very common but inaccurate opinion that sore-mouth in childhood is often produced by the employment of mercury. I never yet saw a sore mouth due to the administration of mercury in any child before the first set of teeth were entirely cut; and never but once out of 70,000 cases which have come under my notice in hospital or dispensary practice, have I seen in children of any age under twelve any affection of the mouth from mercury sufficiently severe to cause me a moment's anxiety.

=Quinsey=, or inflammatory sore-throat, has in it nothing specially peculiar to the child, but occurs at all ages with the same symptoms. It is, however, comparatively rare under twelve years of age, and is almost always less severe in childhood than at or after puberty, while I scarcely remember to have met with it under five years of age. This circumstance attaches special importance to sore-throat in young children, since it will usually be found to betoken the approach of scarlet fever, or of diphtheria, rather than the existence of simple inflammation, or quinsey.

While this fact affords a reason for most scrupulous attention to every case of sore-throat in children, and this in proportion to the tender age of the child, needless alarm is sometimes caused by the appearance on the inflamed tonsils of numerous white specks, which are at once supposed to be diphtheritic. I have already pointed out the distinction between the two conditions when speaking of diphtheria, but the matter is so important that I will repeat what I then said. These spots are not in the form of a uniform white patch or membrane, which, on being removed, leaves the surface beneath red, raw, and often slightly bleeding; but they are rather distinct circular spots, firmly adherent to the tonsil, wiped off with difficulty, and evidently exuding from the openings of little pits, blind pouches, or glands, with which the surface of the tonsil is beset. I do not advise any parent to rest satisfied with his or her judgment on this matter the first time that they notice this appearance; but there are children with whom slight sore-throat is always attended by this condition, and others in whom the tonsils are habitually enlarged, and seldom free from these white spots flecking their surface.

=Enlarged Tonsils.=--I have said that quinsey or acute inflammation of the tonsils is unusual in early childhood; but a sort of chronic inflammation of those glands which leads to their very considerable enlargement is far from uncommon; and is sometimes the cause of very serious discomfort. It is seldom traceable to any acute attack of sore-throat, but usually comes on imperceptibly in children who are feeble or out of health, or takes place slowly during the cutting of the first set of grinding teeth; the irritation which that produces being in some cases its only apparent exciting cause. Not seldom the enlargement has become considerable before it attracts attention; one of the first symptoms that indicate it being the loud snoring of the child during sleep, who is compelled by the obstruction at the back of the nostrils to breathe with its mouth open. The voice at the same time becomes thick, and this and the snoring breathing are both greatly aggravated when the child catches cold.

A greater degree of enlargement of the tonsils occasions deafness from pressure on the passage leading to the internal ear, and is also apt to give rise to a troublesome hacking cough which sometimes excites apprehension lest the child's lungs should be diseased. When still more considerable the enlarged tonsils block up the passage through the nostrils, and air consequently enters the lungs but very imperfectly. The nostrils thus disused become extremely small, narrow, and compressed, the upper jaw does not undergo its proper development, the teeth are crowded and overlap each other, the palate remains narrow and unusually high-arched, and the face assumes something of a bird-like character. Besides this the child grows pigeon-breasted, owing to the lungs not being filled sufficiently at each inspiration to overcome the pressure of the external air on the yielding sides of the chest.

When any considerable enlargement of the tonsils exists, each cold that the child may catch aggravates it, and if diphtheria, scarlatina, or severe sore-throat should occur, the temporary increase of the swelling may become the occasion of serious danger. The question arises, what are the chances that a child whose tonsils are enlarged will outgrow the condition, or when is it necessary to have the enlarged tonsils removed?

It scarcely ever happens that any such enlargement of the tonsils exists in children under six years of age as to call for their removal. There is almost always ground for the hope that after the irritation caused by cutting the first four permanent grinding teeth has completely ceased, the tonsils may return by degrees to their former size. A similar shrinking of the enlarged tonsil sometimes takes place, especially in the boy, at the time of approach to manhood, when the vocal organs undergo full development. This can be counted on, however, only in cases where the tonsils are not of extreme size, and have not undergone frequent attacks of inflammation. Whenever the hearing is habitually dull, and the voice always thick, when cough is frequent, the nostrils narrow, the chest pigeon-breasted, and the child feeble and ill-thriven, removal of the tonsils is absolutely necessary. In cases where the question is doubtful, its decision must turn on whether the tonsils have often been inflamed. So long as their surface is smooth, and their substance soft and elastic, delay is permissible. When their substance is hard, like gristle, and their surface uneven and corrugated, they have undergone such changes that absorption is impossible, and their removal absolutely necessary.

I dwell thus particularly on the question of removal of the tonsils, because there is among many persons an unreasoning dread of the operation, which is entirely devoid of danger, requiring only a few seconds for its performance, and which may even be done under chloroform. The painting tincture of iodine behind the angle of the jaw, or the touching the tonsils with caustic, iodine, alum, tannin, or sweet spirits of nitre are utterly futile proceedings. They diminish the unhealthy and often offensive secretion from the glands which beset the tonsils, and restore the surface to a more healthy condition, but they are absolutely without influence in lessening their size.

Now and then all the symptoms of enlarged tonsils are present, but yet most careful examination fails to discover any increase of their size. When this is the case the symptoms are due to a thickening of the membrane at the back part of the nostrils, often attended with spongy outgrowths from their surface, which obstruct just as completely as enlarged tonsils would do the free entrance of air. It will, in any case where this condition is suspected, be absolutely necessary to seek the advice of some of those gentlemen who make a specialty of diseases of the throat, and who will have the necessary technical dexterity to discover the condition, and to treat it skilfully.

=Abscess at back of the Throat.=--I should pass unnoticed, on account of its rarity, the occasional formation of an abscess at the back of the throat, behind the gullet, interfering both with breathing and with swallowing, but that the description of it in my Lectures once enabled a lady in the wilds of Russia to detect it, to point out the nature of the case to her puzzled doctor, to urge him to open the abscess, and thus to save her child's life.

This abscess may form at any age, sometimes after fever, sometimes without any obvious cause. It shows itself by difficulty in swallowing and breathing, unattended by cough, but accompanied by a sound similar to that of croup, but not so harsh or ringing. The neck is stiff, the head thrown back, and often there is a distinct swelling on one or other side of the neck. The finger introduced into the mouth, and carried over the tongue to the back of the throat, feels there a swelling which projects over the top of the windpipe, and causes the difficulty both in swallowing and breathing. This swelling is the abscess; a prick with the surgeon's lancet lets out the matter, and saves the child.

=Diseases of the Kidneys.=--The kidneys perform very important duties in carrying off from the system a large amount of useless material, and thus supplement in many respects the action of the skin, and the purifying influence which is exercised by the air on the blood, as it passes through the lungs.

It is evident, therefore, that their disorder in any way must be a matter of serious moment, though at the same time the knowledge of the skilled doctor is needed to determine the nature and degree of the ailment from which they are suffering, since that requires an examination of the urine, both chemically and by means of the microscope. My remarks on these diseases must consequently be few and fragmentary.

In the grown person, what is known as Bright's disease is of frequent occurrence, assumes different forms, and depends on various causes. In the child it is comparatively rare, and is scarcely ever met with except as a consequence of a chill, or as a result of scarlatina. In these conditions the kidneys become overfilled with blood or congested, and the congestion may pass into inflammation, by which their structure may be irreparably damaged. Dropsy is the great outward sign of the affection--either slight swelling of the face, eyelids, and ankles, or very great swelling of all the limbs, and even the abundant pouring out of fluid into the belly. The degree of dropsy is, however, by no means an absolute measure of the amount of kidney mischief. It therefore behoves every parent to follow out all directions most scrupulously even in cases of very slight dropsy, in order to guard against the risk of permanent injury to the kidneys being left behind; and especially to remember the liability to the occurrence of dropsy and disease of the kidneys after scarlatina. Any check to the action of the skin while it is peeling or desquamating, as it is termed, is especially liable to be followed by these accidents. To avoid all risks as far as possible, I have been accustomed for many years to insist on a child remaining in bed for one-and-twenty days after the first appearance of the rash in even the mildest case of scarlatina, and I am absolutely sure that it is the height of imprudence ever to neglect this precaution.

It will suffice to mention the fact that diabetes, though very rare, may yet occur in childhood, and that as a rule it is more dangerous in childhood than in the grown person. Whenever a child loses flesh without obvious cause, suffers much from thirst, and at the same time passes urine in greater abundance than in health, the possibility that it may suffer from diabetes must be borne in mind.

Of far greater frequency than any other affection of the kidney is that in which the child passes gravel with the urine, either in the form of a reddish-white sediment, which collects at the bottom of the vessel as the urine cools, or of minute glistening red particles, which resemble grains of cayenne pepper.

These deposits, when abundant in the male child, have a tendency to collect in the bladder, and there to form a stone. This painful disease, too, is so much more frequent in childhood than at a later age, that more than a third--indeed, nearly half--of all the operations for stone performed in English hospitals are done on boys under ten years old.

Even when this grave consequence does not follow the presence of gravel in the kidneys, and its passage into the bladder, it is often accompanied with much suffering. The pain is like that of stomach-ache or colic, the child crying and drawing up its legs on every attempt to pass water, which sometimes is voided only in a few drops at a time, and now and then is completely suppressed for some hours. The very acute form of the ailment seldom occurs, except in infants who inherit from their parents a disposition to gouty or rheumatic affections. In them, however, a trifling cold, slight disorder of the digestion, a state of constipation, or the feverishness and general irritation which sometimes attend on teething, not infrequently produce these deposits and give rise to all these painful symptoms, the deposit disappearing and the pain ceasing so soon as the brief constitutional disturbance subsides.

The very acute attacks seldom occur after the first two years of life, but similar symptoms, though less severe, are by no means unusual in older children, and continue to recur from very trifling causes, especially from errors in diet and disorders of digestion.

In spite of the suffering which for the time attends it, there is no cause for anxiety with reference to the issue of each attack. The warm bath, a castor oil aperient, and soothing medicine soon relieve the pain, and the children return to their former state of health. It is the frequent return of the attack, even in a comparatively mild form, the persistent disposition to the formation of gravel, the remote risk in the case of male children of stone in the bladder, and the habitually imperfect performance of the digestive functions which call for special care. The avoidance of sugar, sweets, and whatever tends to impart acidity to the urine, the maintaining the due action of the skin by wearing flannel, and the judicious use of alkaline remedies, sometimes combined with iron, are the measures on which the doctor is sure to insist.

The difficulty usually encountered in the treatment of these cases arises from the reluctance of the parents to continue for months and years the observance of the necessary rules. It seems so hard to deny their little one the small gratifications in which other children may indulge with impunity; and they fail to realise the heavy penalty, in the shape of gout, rheumatism, gravel, and stone, which in after-life their darling may have to pay for their over-indulgence in his early years.

I will just mention that symptoms similar to those above described, less severe, though more abiding, yet unattended by gravel in the urine, are sometimes produced in little boys by an unnatural narrowness of the end of the passage for the urine. It is well to bear in mind this possible cause of the child's sufferings, and to consult a doctor with reference to it, since he will be able to relieve it by a trivial operation.

=Incontinence of Urine.=--The irritation which this mechanical inconvenience produces sometimes has to do with that troublesome infirmity of some children, who wet the bed at night. This may also be induced by a very acid, and consequently irritating, state of urine, either with or without the appearance in it of gravel. Often, however, it is a result of want of care on the part of the nurse, who neglects to cultivate regular habits in a child; and does not pay attention to the quantity of liquid taken at its last meal. Something, too, is due to the fact that the sleep of a child is deeper than that of the grown person, so that the sensation of want, which would arouse the latter to full consciousness, does not have the same effect on the former. It sometimes happens undoubtedly from mere indolence; and this may always be suspected when a child, otherwise healthy, wets itself not at night only, but also in the daytime. Lastly, it does sometimes occur from muscular feebleness in weakly children, the bladder being unable to bear more than a limited degree of distension.

The accident usually happens either soon after going to bed, when the warmth stimulates the action of the bladder, or towards morning, when the bladder has become full. The posture on the back favours its occurrence very much, and it is therefore of importance that the child should lie on its side when in bed. The good effect of a blister on the lower part of the back as a means of cure was largely due to its forcing the child to lie on its side. This object can be attained, however, in a much kindlier way, by tying half a dozen cotton reels together, and fastening them at the child's back. The habit may also often be broken through by arousing the child in the night, and compelling it to empty its bladder, the hour being first ascertained at which the accident usually happens. For this, however, to be of any real use, the child must be awakened thoroughly; since otherwise it will mechanically, and quite unconsciously, empty its bladder while still asleep. The habit in this case is not in the least overcome; only for the time the bed escapes the wetting. The utensil must therefore be placed on different nights at different parts of the room, so that the child, in order to find it, must have been roused to thorough consciousness.

Lastly, I will add that the cases in which the accident is the result of mere indolence are very rare, and though in such cases strictness may be necessary, yet actual punishment is out of place. As a rule, reward answers much better. A penny, or a threepenny-piece every night that the accident does not happen, and a forfeit of a halfpenny or two pence for every night of misfortune, is a very efficacious help to a cure.

When all these domestic means, persevered in for months, fail to produce any result, medical aid must be called in.

CHAPTER IX.

CONSTITUTIONAL DISEASES.

There remains for consideration a large class of what may be termed constitutional diseases, in which the local ailment is the outcome of a previous disorder of the whole system. These diseases are either acute or chronic. The acute constitutional diseases belong to the class of fevers. These are marked by certain local characteristics, as the swelling of the joints in acute rheumatism, the sore-throat in scarlatina, or the eruption on the skin in smallpox, and their course is more or less strictly limited by distinct periods of increase, acme, and decline. No such rule obtains in the case of consumption, scrofula, and rickets, which are instances of chronic constitutional diseases. In them too the local manifestations of the general disease vary also: the lungs being affected in one case of consumption, the bowels in another; while scrofula may show itself by affection of the glands in one case, by the formation of abscesses in a second, or by disease of the bones in a third.

=Chronic Constitutional Diseases.=--It may perhaps be convenient to study first the chronic constitutional diseases; and afterwards to make a few, and they will be but few, remarks on fevers.

=Consumption= and Scrofula, though similar, are not the same disease. Both, however, depend on some defect in the blood, as the result of which certain materials, incapable of being converted into the natural constituents of the body, are deposited in the substance of different external parts or internal organs. If deposited in small quantities, these materials may be absorbed, as it is termed, that is to say, got rid of, by natural processes, which even now we understand but imperfectly.

If deposited more abundantly, they press upon and gradually spoil the healthy parts in which they are seated, and thereby interfere with the proper performance of their duties. Thus, the deposit of consumption encroaches on the proper substance of the lungs, and so lessens the area in which the blood is exposed to the air and purified: the deposit of scrofula around and in a joint interferes with its powers of movement. Nor is this all; but wherever any deposit has once taken place, it tends especially to increase in that very spot, guided as it were by a certain affinity; and the substance of the previously healthy part is removed as fresh deposit comes to occupy its place. Further, the matter deposited has no power of being changed into healthy substance of lung, or of bone, or of any other part.

A fractured limb may be completely mended; a fluid is poured out around and between the edges of the broken bone; by degrees this hardens, it undergoes changes which convert it into solid bone, and the limb is once more as serviceable as before, though some indications of the fracture may still be perceptible in the texture of the bone itself. Or, a person receives a severe blow on his arm or leg; in course of time the blood which had flowed from the ruptured vessels, and had formed a big bruise, is absorbed, and all is as before the injury was inflicted. If more serious damage has been done, the fibres of some muscles may have been torn, even though the skin remains unbroken. Inflammation is set up, the injured parts die, and are melted down into the matter of an abscess. The abscess discharges itself, its walls contract, the opposite surfaces come into contact, and are welded together again, so that there is no loss of substance, nor anything save a scar on the surface to indicate what has happened.

In the case of the deposits of consumption or scrofula these changes cannot take place. In technical language the matter is said to be incapable of organisation; that is to say, it cannot be transformed by nature's alchemy into anything good or useful. It is rubbish to be got rid of; and the patient's recovery depends on the possibility of getting rid of it. If there is much of it, so as to be removed from the vivifying influence which adjacent living structures still maintain about it, the deposit softens at its centre. This softening gradually extends to the circumference; the mass irritates more and more the parts around it, and where the irritation is greatest the structures yield, and are removed to make a way for its escape, and the patient spits up the contents of the abscess.

But the abscess of the lungs is not like an abscess which follows an injury. It has not formed in the midst of previously healthy parts which are capable of reproducing the original structure; its walls are themselves involved in the disease, and, in accordance with the rule I have already mentioned, 'much will have more,' and the patient goes on spitting up the perpetually renewed contents of the abscess for months or years; until by its gradually increasing size, and the more and more abundant discharge of matter, and further and further destruction of lung-substance, death takes place.

This fatal issue, however, is not invariable. In favourable circumstances, and especially in childhood, the radical constitutional defect may be amended, and with a healthier condition of the blood the unhealthy deposit may cease to take place. The lung-substance, however, with all its curious structure of air-cells and their network of minute vessels where, as in nature's laboratory, the blood receives its due supply of oxygen, is not reproduced. The lung shrinks, the sides of the abscess come together, and by slow degrees a dense material cuts it off from the adjacent healthy structure, but the most complete recovery leaves the patient with his breathing power lessened, and with his vigour consequently more or less impaired.

When the deposit is less considerable, a different change takes place. The material dries by degrees, and is at last converted by a purely chemical change into a hard chalky substance, which in the course of time becomes of more than stony hardness.

Last of all; when the deposit is smallest in quantity, it may be completely got rid of; and a lung in which consumptive disease once existed, may eventually regain perfect soundness.

I have dwelt on these processes as they take place in the lungs; but, allowing for differences of locality, they resemble such as take place elsewhere.

Three important conclusions follow from what has been said.

First. It is only in quite the early stage of consumptive disease that absolutely perfect recovery can be hoped for. There is a euphemism, more amiable than honest, which doctors not seldom make use of, saying that a child's lungs are not diseased, but only tender. They mean by this, that on listening to the chest, they detect such changes in the sounds of breathing as their experience tells them are usually produced in the early stage of consumptive disease of the lungs. If the opinion is confirmed by a second competent medical man, then, and not later, is the time for precautions, for removing the child from school, and for selecting, as far as may be, a suitable winter climate. When the signs of disease are well marked, a reprieve, perhaps a long one, is all that can be confidently reckoned on.

Second. When softening of the consumptive deposit has taken place, of which certain sounds attending breathing are all but conclusive, recovery, even the most complete, always implies loss of a certain amount of lung-substance, and consequently loss of a certain amount of breathing power.

Third, and this is most important, as well as most cheering; consumption, which is at no age the absolutely hopeless disease that it was once supposed to be, admits of far more cheerful anticipations in children than in grown persons, or, for that matter, than in the youth or maiden.

The principal causes of consumptive disease are, hereditary predisposition, and improper feeding in infancy. There are besides two diseases incidental to childhood, and one of them almost peculiar to it, namely typhoid fever and measles, which are more apt than any others to develop a tendency to consumption. During convalescence from either of them, therefore, special care is needed.

In the grown person, consumption almost always attacks the lungs, and this often to the exclusion of other organs. In the child, however, this is not so, and though the lungs are indeed oftener affected than other parts, yet in nearly half of the cases some one or other of the digestive organs is likewise involved, and in about one in seven instances the lungs are free and the digestive organs alone are attacked.

Fever, cough, and wasting are the three sets of symptoms which in some degree or other are always present in consumptive disease of the lungs. The fever in the early stages of consumption is not in general severe; but so long as the evening temperature of a child never exceeds 99° there is no cause for anxiety. On the other hand, if the evening temperature for a week or ten days together always amounts to 100° there is grave presumption that consumptive disease is present. In advanced consumption the evening temperature is constantly 103° to 105° while in the morning it may fall to 101° or 100°

Cough is but rarely absent even in cases where the lungs are but slightly involved, for the irritation of the digestive organs often excites a sympathetic cough, and in these circumstances observation of the evening temperature will often furnish a clue to the right interpretation of the symptoms.

There is a form of cough which is oftenest observed in children between the ages of two and five years, which comes in fits closely resembling those of hooping-cough, and each fit ends in a sort of imperfect 'hoop.' This may depend on a particular form of consumption in which the glands connected with the lungs (the bronchial glands as they are called) are diseased, and not the lung-substance itself. The enlarged glands press on some of the nerves connected with the upper part of the windpipe, and thus occasion the spasmodic cough. Always suspect this when a cough persists for weeks together, not getting rapidly worse as hooping-cough would do, but at the same time not growing better, as would be the case with mild hooping-cough. The doctor on listening to the chest will solve your doubts; the thermometer will help you to decide whether his visit is necessary. I may add that this form of consumptive disease is less serious than that in which the lung-substance is involved.

Consumption sometimes follows bronchitis, especially when a child has been subject to frequent attacks of it. A very slow and imperfect recovery from an attack of bronchitis which had not been specially severe is always a reason for solicitude.

Now and then infants are born with consumptive disease. In that case the lungs are always affected; and the symptoms of fever, cough, and wasting usually show themselves within the first three or four months, and the infants almost invariably die within the year. Now and then, however, an infant thus affected may continue apparently in good health for a few months, and then be suddenly attacked by symptoms of acute inflammation or of severe bronchitis which prove rapidly fatal; and it may be found after death that the acute attack destroyed life because the lungs were already the seat of extensive consumptive disease.

No infant in whose mother's family a predisposition to consumption exists ought to be nursed by its mother, but by a healthy wet nurse; or, if that is impossible, it should be brought up on a milk diet, with but a small admixture of farinaceous food.

There is a form of very rapid, or so-called galloping consumption, which is seldom observed before the age of seven years; generally two or three years later. Its symptoms so closely resemble those of typhoid fever, that it may readily be mistaken for it. I refer to it in order to say that the doctor who mistakes the one for the other can scarcely be regarded as blameworthy; and the mistake is of the less importance since the treatment applicable to the one case would do no harm in the other.

I have already noticed the connection between water on the brain and consumption. It is indeed nothing else than inflammation excited by the presence of the deposit of consumptive matter in the brain or its membranes.

Little has been said hitherto about the wasting which was referred to as one of the characteristics of consumption. When the disease is limited, or nearly so, to the lungs, the wasting is not considerable until the mischief in the chest is far advanced. It must be remembered, however, in order to judge of this, that while in the full-grown man the best sign of health is the persistence for years together of the same weight, the case of the child is different. The child ought to grow in height, and increase in weight, and during these changes the plump infant grows thinner, not by real wasting but by conversion of its fat into bone and muscle. The child is thinner, but is taller and weighs heavier. The only real test therefore of the condition of the child is afforded by its increase in height and in weight. One need not be solicitous about the child who increases in height, and maintains his previous weight, nor about him who while he does not grow yet becomes heavier; but the child who neither gains in weight, nor in height, or who loses weight out of proportion to his increased height, is in a condition that warrants anxiety. I have long been accustomed, in the case of children whose parents were resident in India, to instruct those who have charge of them to send every three months a statement of the height and weight of the children, as the best evidence of their state of health.

=Consumptive Disease of the Bowels.=---Consumptive disease sometimes invades the whole system from the very first, while in other instances it attacks from the outset the organs of digestion, and continues throughout to affect them chiefly, and loss of flesh is then one of its earliest symptoms. In instances where there is a strong family predisposition to the disease, consumption of the bowels or mesenteric disease, or disease of the glands of the bowels, all three popular names for the affection, sometimes shows itself at the time of weaning. In the majority of cases, however, it comes on later, after the completion of teething, and between the age of three and ten years. Indigestion such as I have already spoken of sometimes precedes it, with the irregular condition of bowels, and the patchy state of the tongue. But this is by no means constant, scarcely I think general; and not infrequently momentary, causeless, colicky pains precede for a short time any other symptom. In a few weeks after their occurrence, sometimes indeed independently of them, the appetite fails, or becomes capricious; the bowels begin to act irregularly, being alternately constipated and relaxed; and the motions are unnatural in character, being, for the most part, dark, loose, and slimy. Sometimes indeed, they are solid, and then often white, as if from complete inactivity of the liver, and sometimes half-liquid, frothy, and like yeast. One peculiarity which they always present, be their other characters what they may, is their extreme abundance, quite out of proportion to the quantity of food taken, and due to their admixture with the unhealthy secretions from the bowels. The child next becomes restless and feverish at night, its thirst is considerable, and the colicky pains become both more severe and more frequent. Sometimes the stomach grows very irritable, and the food taken is occasionally vomited, while the tongue, in the early stages of the affection, continues for the most part clean and moist, and except that it is often unnaturally red deviates but little from its appearance in health. Next comes a change in the condition of the belly, the date of which varies considerably. It becomes larger than natural, owing to the filling of the bowels with wind, but at the same time it is tense and tender on pressure-- two points of great importance to be noticed, and the glands in the groin, which in a healthy child cannot be felt, become enlarged, and are felt and perhaps even seen like tiny beans under the skin.

As in other forms of consumptive disease, so here the progress from bad to worse seldom goes on uninterruptedly. Pauses take place in its course, though each time they become shorter; and signs of amendment now and then appear, but they too promise less and less with each return. The child wastes rapidly; is always more or less feverish; the abdomen is constantly tender, but does not in general go on increasing in size; the pains become more frequent and more severe, and the bowels are almost always habitually relaxed. Life is sometimes cut short by the lungs becoming affected, but when this is not the case the patient may linger on for weeks, or months, or even for two or three years, until, worn to a skeleton, death at last takes place from exhaustion.

Much apprehension is often needlessly excited in the minds of parents, with reference to any child whose digestion is imperfect, who loses flesh, and has a large abdomen; and the words mesenteric disease, sometimes uttered thoughtlessly by the doctors, seem to them to seal their little one's doom. Now, first of all, it must be remembered that mesenteric disease, due to consumption, plays but a very small part in the production of the symptoms just described, but that the covering and the lining of the bowels are chiefly involved. Next, enlargement of the mesenteric glands and disorder of their functions take place from many causes other than consumption. They are always more or less enlarged in typhoid fever; they become enlarged when irritated by unwholesome food in infancy, or they may swell in the course of chronic indigestion. In all these cases too, the glands in the groin may be enlarged by sympathy, and this without the existence of any actual abiding disease. A big abdomen is, of itself, no evidence of it, nor even when associated with indigestion and frequent stomach-ache; but when to these you add abiding tenderness, and an evening temperature always at least one degree above that in the morning, there is every reason to fear that consumptive disease has attacked the organs of digestion.

Even then, however, there is no ground for despair; for, while consumptive disease in any form is less seldom recovered from in childhood than in after-life, such recovery oftener takes place in cases of affection of the digestive organs than when the disease is seated elsewhere.

=Scrofula.=--With this word of comfort I leave the subject of consumption, and pass to that of the allied disease scrofula. Briefly stated, two of the great differences between it and consumption are that scrofula is almost entirely limited to childhood and youth, while consumption may occur at any age; and next, that while scrofula attacks the bones and the glands, the skin and the membranes adjacent to it, consumption has its seat in the lungs, the brain, and the internal organs.

Scrofulous diseases of the bones come so exclusively under the observation of the surgeon, that I do not feel myself competent to say anything about them. I would however warn all parents to be very much alive to the importance of noticing the early symptoms of any such diseases, as shown by slight lameness, complaint of pain in the back, or difficulty in moving the hand or arm, or in turning the head or bending the neck. They may be but temporary accidents, due to cold, or to slight muscular rheumatism, or to some sprain not noticed at the time; but they may also be signs of the commencement of scrofulous disease of some bone; and in no disease whatever is early judicious treatment of greater value, or the result of neglect less remediable.

Besides these graver ailments which seldom appear until after the time of infancy has passed, there are others of a less serious nature which often show themselves within the first year of life. One of these consists in the formation beneath the skin of numerous small lumps of a rounded form, and of the size of a kidney-bean, slightly movable, and not tender. By degrees such lumps become adherent to the skin, the surface of which above them grows red, they project slightly above it, and at last open by a small circular aperture, discharge a little matter, and then subside. They collapse and disappear; a slight depression and a degree of lividity of the skin mark for a considerable time the situation they had occupied. I refer to them, because while they are a sign of a scrofulous constitution, which may require special care in diet and preparations of iron and cod-liver oil, they are best left absolutely alone--neither poulticed nor lanced. The same principle of non-intervention applies equally to the swellings which sometimes form on two or three of the fingers in infancy, not involving the joints but producing great thickening and a hard swelling around the bone. These swellings disappear by degrees as the constitutional vigour improves, and this is especially promoted by a long stay at the seaside; but they tend, if the health fails, to affect the bones themselves, and thus to occasion deformities of the hand.

Glandular swelling, discharges from the ear, offensive secretion from the nose, and in female children, even of very tender age, a discharge of whites, are all common signs of a scrofulous constitution, and all tedious and troublesome. They all, however, are very much under the influence of judicious medical treatment. It must at the same time be borne in mind that none of these ailments admit of what may be called active treatment. There are no royal means of dispersing scrofulous glands, or of curing discharges from the ear, or of doing away with the offensive smell which in some cases proceeds from the nostrils. Fresh air, suitable diet, preparations of iron, residence at the seaside, and sea-bathing, measures directed to improve the general health, are of chief value, and without them local treatment is of small avail.

A few words, however, may with propriety be added with reference to the local treatment of the minor ailments to which I have just referred.

No local application is of use in the scrofulous swellings of the fingers. Tincture of iodine, indeed, may be painted over them when quite small, while at the same time the joints are kept quiet by a small gutta-percha splint. When they become considerable, iodine is useless; and even if matter forms in the swelling it is much better to let it make its way out by a small opening spontaneously than to make a puncture with a lancet, since the edges of the wound would not heal, and the risk of the disease affecting the bone would be increased.

The glandular swellings of the neck or about the lower jaw are likewise best let alone, or merely covered with a layer of cotton wool, stitched inside a piece of oiled silk to maintain a uniform temperature. If they become suddenly painful and more swollen, a cooling lotion of Goulard water and spirits of wine, constantly applied, will reduce the swelling and lessen the discomfort. When stationary, a mild iodine ointment may be smeared over the gland at bedtime, and covered with oiled silk. Applications of iodine, however, need careful watching, for sometimes they over-irritate the gland, and cause an abscess. If the gland were out of sight there would be no objection to this, which would probably be a rapid mode of getting rid of the swelling; but the scar left behind, if the abscess burst or were opened, is an objection when the swelling is situated in the neck or at the jaw.

If the skin over the top of the swelling becomes red, and its substance begins to feel soft, then, but not till then, it is desirable to apply a warm poultice constantly. At the same time the progress must be daily watched by the doctor, in order that he may seize the proper moment to make a small puncture and let out the matter. The small cut leaves a less puckered scar than the natural opening. The subsequent management of the case must be superintended by the doctor.

Offensive discharge from the nostrils does not depend, in by far the majority of cases, on disease of the bones, but on an unhealthy condition of their lining membrane. It is exceedingly obstinate and difficult of cure, is four times more frequent in girls than in boys, and unfortunately often lasts into womanhood, and continues even when the general health is perfect.

Much may be done to abate the annoyance by diligent sniffing up the nostrils some weak disinfectant; or by regularly irrigating the nostrils by means of a simple apparatus, to be obtained from any instrument-maker. In spite of this, however, it is often necessary to introduce a little plug of cotton wool dipped in the fluid some distance up the nostrils, with a thread attached by which it can be withdrawn, and a fresh one substituted twice a day.

The discharge of whites is sometimes very troublesome, and apt to return from the commencement of teething up even to womanhood. It is a mere sign of debility, usually also connected with a scrofulous habit, but has no further or graver meaning. Locally, constant cold ablution by means of a sponge held above the child, not touching it, is the great remedy, and this may have to be repeated every hour or two if the case is severe. Astringent lotions of different kinds may be used in the same manner; while care must be taken that the child's drawers are large and loose, so as not to irritate her when sitting. General treatment, however, sea air and sea bathing are especially in these cases the great remedy.

It must not be forgotten that all these ailments have a special tendency to recur; and that when people say 'Dr. A. or Dr. B. did the child good for the time, but this or that symptom returned as soon as the treatment was discontinued,' as though this were the doctor's fault, they are unjust; for the tendency to return of every form of scrofulous disease is one of the great characteristics of the malady. Patience and perseverance on the parents' part, even for months and years, are often as much needed as skill on the part of the doctor.

One more remark may not be out of place. Some persons have an impression that there is something specially shameful in scrofulous disease, and while they will readily admit the existence of a consumptive tendency in their family, they almost resent the suggestion that their child's ailment is scrofulous. For this prejudice there is absolutely no foundation. There is no more reason for connecting scrofula in a child with any antecedent wrong-doing on the part of its progenitors, than there is for attaching that idea to the red hair or black eyes which a child may have in common with the rest of its family.

=Rickets.=--We sometimes see, especially in the poorer quarters of a great city, persons dwarfed in stature, with large hands, bowed legs, bent arms, swollen wrists and ankles, walking with an awkward gait, though usually holding themselves remarkably upright, with the face of a grown person on the body of a child, and we know that they suffered from rickets when young.

Rickets is essentially a disease of childhood, and of early childhood, in which proper bone-formation does not take place, the soft material, or gristle, which should turn to bone, remaining long in the soft state. When, therefore, the child begins to walk, or to use its limbs, they bend under the weight of the body, or under their own weight, and with every slight movement which its feeble muscular power enables it to make. It does more, however, than interfere with the hardening of the limbs: it arrests growth to a great degree, interferes with development, retards teething, postpones the closure of the open part of the head, or fontanelle, weakens constitutional vigour, and impairs muscular power. To this feeble muscular power it is due that the child cannot make the effort to fill its lungs completely, and hence the pressure of the external air forces the soft ribs inwards, and gives to the chest the peculiar form of pigeon-breast. In the course of time the delayed bone-formation takes place, and the bones themselves become as hard as ivory, but the limbs do not straighten, and the deformity produced in infancy is but confirmed in after-life.

The greater degrees of rickets are scarcely ever seen among the children of the wealthier classes, but over-crowded and ill-ventilated nurseries, cots from which the air is well-nigh shut out by closed sides and overhanging curtains; injudicious feeding, with undue preponderance of farinaceous food, often produce its slighter forms. I never yet saw rickets in a child while brought up exclusively at its mother's breast.

The slighter forms of rickets show themselves in a tardy closure of the infant's head, which sweats profusely when the child is laid down to sleep; in big wrists, which contrast with the attenuated arms; in a general limpness of the whole body, and a bowing of the back under the weight of the head, which bends as a green stick would bend if a weight were placed upon it. They are further marked by backwardness in teething, and by the irregular order in which the teeth appear, and, further, by the peculiar narrowness of the chest, and by what has been termed the beading of the ends of the ribs: little round prominences due to a heaping up of gristle just where the ribs join on to the breastbone, marking the spots at which the tardy bone-making has come to a standstill.

Children who bear these stamps of rickets are far more apt than others to suffer from spasmodic croup, and in them it is also specially likely to be severe and to be accompanied by convulsions. They will also be more liable than others to attacks of bronchitis, they will suffer more during teething, they will be often constipated, and will be troubled by various forms of indigestion. Now and then, too, they will have causeless attacks of feverishness lasting for a few days, or for two or three weeks, attended with general tenderness of the surface, and a disposition to perspiration, which brings no relief but serves only to weaken.

It is true that these symptoms do not often become immediately dangerous to life, though spasmodic croup and bronchitis both have their perils; but they interfere with health, and growth, and good looks, and cheerfulness, and quick intelligence.

If mothers would but ask themselves the real signification of these symptoms, and change the conditions which surround the child, and alter their mode of feeding it, they would many and many a time be spared the heart-ache of seeing their little ones grow up weakly, ugly, ill-thriven.

Unfortunately, it is so much easier to give cod-liver oil and iron than to turn the best spare room into a night nursery, and to uglify the cot by taking away the curtains which made it so pretty, and to give up some of the pleasures of society in order to superintend the preparation of the baby's food; that the doctor is called in to correct by drugs the evil which drugs cannot reach. Iron and cod-liver oil are very useful in the second place; fresh air, good ventilation, and a wise diet must always occupy the first.

=Acute Constitutional Diseases.=--It still remains for us to glance rapidly at the characters of the acute constitutional diseases, all of which belong, as has already been stated, to the class of fevers. Of them all but two are contagious--that is to say, are capable of being communicated directly from person to person. They are likewise infectious, or, in other words, articles of bedding or clothes which have been worn by the sick, retain a something--an exhalation from the breath, an emanation from the skin, or a secretion from the bowels--which may reproduce the same disease in a person previously healthy.

To this contagious and infectious property there are two exceptions; the one is furnished by acute rheumatism, or rheumatic fever, the other by intermittent fever, or ague.

=Rheumatic Fever.=--The main features of rheumatic fever are the same at all ages. Fever, pain in the limbs, swelling of the joints, sweats unattended by that relief which usually accompanies abundant action of the skin in fevers, are its characteristics. In the child all these symptoms are usually less even than in the adult. The swelling of the joints in particular is less considerable, and both the pain and the swelling are apt to wander from one to another joint, or to a different limb, instead of remaining fixed as they do in the grown person for several days in the same joint, even though fresh joints may be implicated in the course of the disease.

These circumstances tend to make people look on rheumatic fever in the child too often as a comparatively trivial ailment; and this not only because the suffering which attends the disease is slighter, but because its duration is also shorter. But there is one fact which forbids this low estimate of its importance, and that is the great tendency to affection of the heart even in cases of comparatively mild rheumatism in the child; while in the grown person there is a direct relation between the general severity of the rheumatic symptoms and the liability of the heart to be involved. I have already stated that nine out of ten of all cases of heart disease in early life, not due to original malformation, are of rheumatic origin, and further that heart disease comes on in the course of four out of five cases of rheumatic fever in the child, slight as well as severe. It seldom occurs before the third or fourth day of the illness, so that if parents take the alarm at the very outset, it is usually though not invariably possible for the doctor by judicious treatment to anticipate and to prevent its occurrence, or at any rate greatly to control its progress.

Every threatening of rheumatism, therefore, is to be watched with the most anxious care, since so serious a complication as disease of the heart may accompany extremely slight general symptoms. It is wise too, to place any child in whom general feverish symptoms come on at once under medical observation, for though it does not usually happen, yet it does sometimes occur, that rheumatic inflammation attacks the heart before any other local signs of the malady have manifested themselves. It is scarcely necessary to add that tenfold precautions are needed when rheumatism has once occurred, since the liability to its return is very great, and the heart which escaped in the first attack may suffer in the second; or the comparatively small mischief done the first time may become an incurable disorder.

=Ague.=--Intermittent fever or ague is very rare in childhood in London; or at any rate it is very rare among children of the wealthier classes. I believe it is everywhere rarer among children than among grown persons, probably because they are as a rule less exposed to those malarious influences which produce it. In the child it generally takes the form of tertian ague, that is to say the attack recurs every second day; one day of freedom intervening between two attacks.

The three stages of shivering, heat, and sweating are less marked in the child than in the grown person, and this indistinctness of its symptoms is greater in proportion to the tenderer age of the child. Shivering is scarcely ever well-marked, a condition of unaccountable depression usually taking its place, while once or twice I have known convulsions occur which gave rise to the apprehension that disease of the brain existed. The hot stage is long, and passes off gradually without the profuse perspiration that occurs in the grown person, and the child even between the attacks is almost always more or less ailing.

A first and even a second attack may puzzle not the parents only, but also the doctor; but after the symptoms have returned a few times, the child being neither better nor worse in the intervals, it becomes evident that no serious disease is impending. The risk of an overhasty conclusion is that the depression and disturbance of the nervous system may be supposed to imply the existence of brain disease; and lead to unsuitable treatment, instead of the administration of quinine, which nine times out of ten proves a specific for ague. The rapid increase of temperature in the attack, and its equally rapid subsidence afterwards, will, if carefully noted, preserve from error.

There is much that is obscure with reference to the nature both of rheumatic and intermittent fever. They differ from other fevers not only by being neither contagious nor infectious but also by their readiness to return, while a single attack of any of the others furnishes a guarantee, and often a complete guarantee, against its recurrence. In addition to these peculiarities, the fevers of which I have now to speak are characterised by running a certain definite course, being accompanied by certain peculiar appearances on the surface (generally rashes on the skin, whence their name of eruptive fevers); being attended each with its own peculiar dangers, and all having a tendency to what is termed epidemic prevalence; that is to say to occur one year, and without obvious cause with vastly greater frequency than in other years.

=Mumps.=--It has been questioned whether that painful but not dangerous ailment the mumps, ought or ought not to be classed with these fevers. I think it should, for it is contagious, infectious, runs a fairly definite course, is attended with invariable external appearances, often prevails epidemically, and one attack preserves in most instances from a second.

It very seldom befalls children under seven years of age, and is more frequent in early youth than in childhood. It sets in with the ordinary symptoms of a cold, which are followed in about twenty-four hours by stiffness of the neck, and pain about the lower jaw, which is increased by speaking or swallowing. At the same time a swelling appears, sometimes on one side sometimes on both of the lower jaw, and increases very rapidly so as to occasion great disfigurement of the face. The swelling goes on to increase, and to become more tense, attended with more head-ache, fever, and discomfort for some forty-eight hours, but then it begins to lessen, and the general illness subsides rapidly, though the enlarged gland, for that is the cause of the swelling, sometimes does not return to its natural size for a week, ten days, or more; and now and then, though very rarely, an abscess forms, which is both tedious and troublesome.

The treatment suitable for a severe common cold, together with the constant application of a warm poultice to the swollen gland, is all that is usually required, though the doctor's help is often needed to relieve the suffering which for the first day or two in many instances attends the ailment.

=Typhoid Fever.=--There is no question as to the place which should be occupied by typhoid fever, smallpox, measles, and scarlatina, for all belong to the class of eruptive fevers. They are all specific diseases, each due to its own peculiar poison, and not capable of being produced by any mere unsanitary conditions, though such may aggravate their severity and facilitate their spread.

The belief in the special character of each of these diseases has received strong confirmation from the researches of the eminent Frenchman, M. Pasteur, and others who have followed in his track. They have discovered in the blood and other secretions, and in some of the tissues both of men and animals, minute microscopic organisms which differ in their characters in different diseases. Experiment has further shown that in some mysterious way these organisms are the cause of these diseases, for on inoculating animals with them the peculiar disease of which each was the accompaniment, and no other, was reproduced in the inoculated animal.

As far as our knowledge goes at present then, we are forced to regard each of these as a separate disease, measles never passing into scarlatina, nor that into smallpox, but each, whether slight or severe, retaining throughout its distinct character.

We have already seen how, in the course of various diseases, the pulse is quickened, and the temperature raised, constituting that state which we commonly call fever, but as the local ailment subsides the fever disappears. There is, apart from smallpox, measles, and the other so-called eruptive fevers, only one real essential fever commonly met with in childhood, and that is what the doctors call typhoid fever. The name, from the similarity of sound to typhus, from which, however, it is essentially different, has long been a name of terror in the nursery, and all sorts of epithets have been substituted for it, as gastric fever, and infantile remittent fever, and so on. Name it as you may, the fever is one and the same with the typhoid fever, which one hears of as prevailing constantly in many continental cities, and proving dangerous and fatal in any district almost in direct relation to the neglect of drainage and of proper sanitary precautions.

It is extremely rare in infancy, though I saw it once in a babe eight months old, and is comparatively seldom met with before the age of five years. From five to ten years old it is more frequent than from ten to fifteen, but it is consolatory to know that it is less fatal in early childhood than at any subsequent time of life, and that cases of such exceedingly mild character that the child's condition can be more properly described as ailing rather than ill, are then far from uncommon. The symptoms, however, are in all instances similar in kind, though widely varying in degree, and the duration of the fever is, as nearly as may be, three weeks. By this it is not meant that at three weeks' end the child who has had typhoid fever is well again, but only that the temperature, which had hitherto been high, and always higher at night than in the morning, has subsided, that the skin has become less dry, the tongue slightly moist, the intelligence more clear, that the fever has run its course. For the first week or ten days, the symptoms have probably become every day more grave; and for the next ten the doctor could find no better consolation than the assurance--happy if he could give it--that the condition was not worse, but that you must have patience, for the time for improvement had not yet arrived. If the attack has been severe, the child will be left greatly exhausted, sadly emaciated, and suffering from the effects of that ulceration of the bowels which accompanies the fever, and from which life may still be in imminent danger. But the fire is quenched; the question is no longer how to put out the conflagration, but how to repair the mischief it has caused.

When mild, the disease usually comes on very gradually, the child loses its cheerfulness, the appearance of health leaves it, the appetite fails, and the thirst becomes troublesome; in the daytime it is listless and fretful, and drowsy towards evening, but the nights are often restless, and the slumber broken and unrefreshing. The skin is hotter, and almost always drier than natural, or if there is any perspiration, it comes on at irregular times, lasts but an hour or two and brings no refreshing. The thermometer will quite, in the early days, solve all doubt as to the nature of the case. In the morning the thermometer will be natural, or nearly so, but at seven o'clock in the evening it will have risen to 101?or 102? and will continue so during the early part of the unquiet night. After midnight it will begin to fall, and by six o'clock in the morning, or even earlier, will have regained its natural standard. There is no other disease but typhoid fever, and now and then some forms of galloping consumption, in which these oscillations of temperature take place regularly. Other symptoms attend typhoid fever besides these, and serve to stamp upon it its distinctive character. The bowels are usually loose, or if not, a moderate aperient acts on them excessively, the evacuations being loose, often watery, of a light yellow-ochrey colour. The abdomen is full, the bowels being more or less distended with wind, sometimes tender, especially at the right side, and both tender and painful in all cases where the disease is severe. Towards the end of the first, or at the latest by the middle of the second week, small rose-red spots or pimples appear on the abdomen, sometimes also on the chest and back. They disappear for the moment if pressure is made on them, but reappear the moment the pressure is withdrawn. Now and then they are numerous, and sometimes two or three successive crops appear, the old ones fading as the others show themselves; but in childhood they are often scanty, though whether few or many, they are the external characteristic of the disease just as the rash is in scarlatina or measles.

Whenever a child of whatever age begins without obvious cause to lose appetite and health, to become feverish, with marked increase of temperature towards evening for several days together, and more or less disposition to diarrh[oe]a, it is all but absolutely certain that the child has contracted typhoid fever.

When the disease comes on gradually, it seldom becomes dangerous, though until the end of the first week there is always considerable uncertainty on this point. The amount of diarrh[oe]a and the degree of disorder of the brain, as shown by restlessness, delirium, and stupor are the measure of the gravity of any case. There is, however, scarcely any disease from which even when most severe recovery so often takes place in childhood, and this not as persons so often imagine from some critical occurrence but by a process of gradual amendment. The first signs of amendment, too, may be taken as giving almost certain promise of complete recovery; but it is well to bear in mind that there is no disease of early life in which the mental faculties, though time brings them back at length uninjured, remain so long in a state of feebleness and torpor as in typhoid fever. Though the first signs of improvement, too, are very seldom deceptive, yet the patient's convalescence is almost always slow, and interrupted by many fluctuations.

Though contagious, still typhoid fever is far less directly contagious than measles or scarlatina. It seems as if with this disease, just as with cholera, the contagious element were present in its most active form in the discharges from the bowels. These should therefore be disinfected by carbolic acid or some other disinfectant immediately; and should never be emptied in a closet used by other members of the family, and more particularly by children. Special precautions also should be taken with the bed-linen, and night-dresses of the patient; and it must be remembered that wise precautions have nothing in common with exaggerated alarm. One more hint will not be out of place. In typhoid fever, and still more in the highly contagious measles and scarlatina, the person who sleeps in the patient's room is much more likely to contract the disease than she who sits up and watches at night keeping wide awake. Whoever takes charge of a fever patient during the night should therefore sit up and watch, not lie down and doze, and this not for the patient's sake only, but for her own.

It can scarcely be necessary to say that in every, even the mildest, attack of typhoid fever the attendance of the doctor is needed from first to last. He may come every day, and may daily do nothing but merely watch. The disease will run its course, the greatest skill cannot cut it short, though now and then instead of lasting for three or even four weeks it comes to an end spontaneously in fourteen days. Skilled watching is what the competent doctor gives. You would not despise or underestimate the pilot's skill, who steered your barque through a dangerous sea in smoothest water, because he knew each hidden rock or unseen quicksand on which but for his guidance you might have made shipwreck.

=Small-pox.=--At the present day, thanks to vaccination, and to re-vaccination, small-pox is rarely met with in the well-to-do classes of society, though it is not yet a century ago since it found its victims not only among the poor, but among the highest in the land. It does, however, occur sometimes after vaccination, and sometimes, though very rarely, an attack of small-pox fails to furnish an absolute guarantee against the occurrence of a second.

Small-pox, unmodified by previous vaccination, sets in in the child with violent sickness; vomiting, sometimes recurring frequently for forty-eight hours, with much depression, or even stupor; in some instances even actual convulsions, and fever; but neither with the sore-throat of scarlatina, nor with the sneezing, cough, and running at the nose of measles. At the end of from forty-eight to sixty hours, an eruption of pimples appears on the face, forehead, forearms and wrists, whence it extends to the body and the lower limbs. They are reddish in colour, rather pointed in form, and at first scarcely raised above the surface; so that the eruption looks at first like the very early eruption of measles; though the tiny pimples felt as if beneath the skin serve even then to distinguish the one disease from the other. In another forty-eight hours the character of the pimples has changed into that of little vesicles or pocks, depressed instead of pointed at their centre, and containing a little watery milky fluid. They next enlarge, and become once more prominent at their centre as they fill more and more with fluid, which becomes thicker, yellowish-white--looks like, and indeed is, matter. Four or five days are occupied with this process; the matter in the pocks then begins to dry, and scabs to form, which gradually by the end of another week drop off, and leave the skin spotted with red or even scarred if the pocks went deep enough to destroy the skin, and to leave the indelible marks, the so-called pitting of small-pox.

The danger of the disease is in childhood the nervous disorder at the outset, and then the exhaustion produced by the so-called maturation of the pocks when the thin watery fluid changes to the thicker matter, and depresses the patient in the same way as he would be depressed by an enormous abscess.

The first outbreak of the eruption is followed always by a most remarkable abatement in the disturbance of the constitution, and for three or four days, even though the eruption is abundant, the patient may seem so well that it is almost impossible to realise the imminent peril to which he will be exposed in a few days' time.

=Inoculation and Vaccination.=--The danger of small-pox is in direct proportion to the abundance of the eruption; and the great advantage of inoculation for the small-pox consisted in the much scantier eruption which followed it, as compared with that which commonly took place in the natural small-pox.

The same advantage in a greater degree is obtained by vaccination, even in the exceptional instances in which it fails to render the person altogether insusceptible to the disease.

The great advantage which inoculation secured was counterbalanced in great measure by the fact that it always maintained small-pox rife throughout the whole country, and that consequently all who either had neglected inoculation, or young children on whom, on account of their tender age, it had not yet been practised, were more than ever exposed to constant risk of infection.

This very real danger led to the almost unanimous welcome which the practice of vaccination received towards the end of the last century, since it was hoped that by it not only would the risk attending small-pox be lessened, and the disease when it did occur be even milder in character than inoculated small-pox, but that small-pox itself would eventually be extirpated.

These anticipations have not hitherto been fully realised; but the good effected by vaccination has been such as to render it, in the opinion of nearly everyone qualified to form an opinion on the subject, one of the greatest boons ever conferred on the human race.

Small-pox, like other eruptive fevers, has the peculiarity of occurring for the most part only once in a person's life. We do not know in the least on what this protecting influence depends. We know the fact, but are the less able to offer an explanation, since there are other constitutional diseases, such as gout and rheumatism, in which the local symptoms are equally the outcome of previous constitutional disorder, where exactly the opposite rule obtains, and in which their occurrence does but increase the liability to their return.

The protective power is apparently possessed by the mild form of the disease communicated by inoculation as much as by the severer form of small-pox which is contracted by direct contagion or infection. This knowledge has been applied in the treatment of some of the diseases of animals, and it has been found in the case of the so-called small-pox in sheep (a disease which, however, is quite distinct from human small-pox) that while one in two of the animals who contracted it in the ordinary way died, death took place in only three per cent, or not one in thirty, of those in whom it was produced by inoculation; and the inoculated sheep were thereby safeguarded from subsequent attacks as completely as the others.

This knowledge was more recently applied by the distinguished Frenchman whom I have already mentioned, M. Pasteur, in the case of a fatal pestilence among sheep in many parts of France, known by the name of charbon. The inoculated sheep died, however, in such large numbers, though in a somewhat smaller proportion than those who had been directly infected, that he found it necessary to weaken the matter which he employed by admixture with other innocuous materials. This experiment, however, again yielded unsatisfactory results; slight symptoms of the disease were produced, but the protection thus afforded was inadequate and uncertain. Some few resisted the disease, but others contracted it and died. With that clear insight which constitutes genius, M. Pasteur next tried the experiment of inoculating the sheep first with a weak matter which produced but slight symptoms, but at the same time enabled the animal to support a second inoculation with a stronger matter; and this second inoculation enabled them to bear, unharmed, subsequent exposure to the disease. A grateful country has given a pension, and conferred well-merited honours on the man who has preserved their flocks from pestilence, but whom the silly sentimentality of the anti-vivisectionists in England would have mulcted in a fine, and, if possible, have sent to prison.

That weakening of the poisonous element which Pasteur strove to attain by art, is already provided by nature in the cow-pox. The cow-pox is nothing else than small-pox modified in character, diminished in severity by passing through the system of the animal; but giving, when introduced into the system, a safeguard against natural small-pox at least as complete as that furnished by the inoculated disease.

More than 70,000 children have come under my observation, either in hospital or in private practice; and I need not say that a physician having much consulting practice sees far more than the average of unusual and severe cases. Twice, and only twice, I have seen infants die from vaccination, and in both instances death took place from erysipelas beginning at the puncture. The one case I saw twice in consultation with the family practitioner. The other which I watched throughout was that of a little boy, the fifth child of a nobleman of high rank, both his parents being perfectly healthy. He was vaccinated by the family doctor in the country, direct from the arm of another perfectly healthy infant, from whom ten other infants were vaccinated immediately afterwards. The little boy was seized with convulsions within twenty-four hours, and almost at the same time erysipelas appeared on the punctured arm. The erysipelas extended rapidly, convulsions returned more than once, and on the fourth day from the vaccination the child died. One of the other children vaccinated at the same time died in the country in the same manner; all the others passed through vaccination regularly, and without a single bad symptom. I have no explanation to offer; this case stands by itself just as do those of death from the sting of a bee or death from cutting a corn.

That some people die of other diseases since the introduction of vaccination, is undoubtedly true, for many of those who would have died in early infancy of small-pox are cut off later by measles or bronchitis, or die during teething; since it is obvious that vaccination does not protect against any other disease than small-pox.

That protection, indeed, is not absolute, nor was the protection afforded by inoculation absolute; but small-pox after vaccination, even when it does occur, is very rarely severe, and still more seldom fatal.

There seems good reason for believing that the protecting power of vaccination tends to diminish with the lapse of time; though apparently this is not always the case, nor can any direct statement be made as to the conditions which favour this in one case, or prevent it in another. As a matter of fact, however, we do know that such a tendency does exist, and that this tendency calls for the repetition of vaccination from time to time; such re-vaccination carefully performed being as nearly as possible an absolute guarantee against small-pox. All persons engaged as nurses or attendants at the Small-Pox Hospital during the past thirty-two years, have been vaccinated or re-vaccinated before entering on their duties, and during this period not a single case of the disease has occurred among the whole staff. The experience of other small-pox hospitals for a shorter period is identical. As far as we know, every seventh year is a reasonable interval at which re-vaccination should be performed.

One great cause of the failure of the protective power of vaccination is the unintelligent and careless manner in which it is too often performed, especially among the poor. To this same cause it is also due that in some cases of almost infinite rarity one special constitutional disease has been known to be communicated. I have never seen such a case, but I know there are such. They are, however, no more a reason against vaccination than the occasional death from an overdose of opium is a reason against the use of that drug.

To avoid any risk of this kind, and also with the idea that the power of the vaccine matter may have become weakened by transmission through many thousands of persons, vaccination direct from the calf has been introduced of late years, especially in America and on the Continent. The time, however, that has as yet elapsed is scarcely sufficient to test the comparative preservative power of this as compared with vaccination from the human subject. Its immediate local effects are somewhat more severe; I do not know any reason why its influence should not be equally abiding.

There is absolutely no foundation for the idea that scrofula, consumption, or any similar disease can be transmitted by vaccination. In some infants, whose skin is very delicate, and especially in those, some members of whose family have been liable to eruptions on the skin, vaccination has seemed to act as an irritant, and to give occasion to an eruption, or aggravate an eruption already existing. Such cases, however, are not frequent, and the eruption is not more troublesome than those which often appear in teething children. The occurrence of actual erysipelas around the puncture, while very dangerous, is, as I have already stated, of excessive rarity.

A thoroughly dispassionate review of the whole subject appears to me to warrant the following conclusions:--

1st. That vaccination, though not a perfect guarantee against small-pox, diminishes immensely the risk of its occurrence; and that by periodical revaccination, this guarantee is rendered all but absolute.

2nd. That a very large proportion of the failures of vaccination are due to its careless and imperfect performance.

3rd. That to such careless performance and to the introduction of the blood and not of the vaccine matter alone, from one child to another are due the extremely rare instances in which one special disease has been transmitted by vaccination.

4th. That there is absolutely no evidence of the transmission of scrofula, consumption, or any similar disease by vaccination.

5th. That vaccination direct from the calf appears to present some decided advantages; but it has not yet been practised for a sufficient time to admit of a comparison between its preservative power and that of vaccination from one child to another.

6th. That in either case it is expedient that vaccination be performed within the first three months after birth, so as to avoid the irritation of teething which is unfavourable to successful vaccination, and also because the disposition to those skin diseases which vaccination tends to aggravate is never so considerable before the age of three months as it becomes subsequently.

Even when vaccination fails to protect against small-pox it tends to produce a modified and so much milder form of the disease, that while one patient died out of every two in the Homerton Small Pox Hospital who had the disease naturally, the deaths were only one in four of those who had been imperfectly vaccinated, and one in forty-three of those whose arms bore evidence of perfectly good and successful vaccination.

The influence of previous vaccination often scarcely shows itself in the stage which precedes the appearance of the eruption of small-pox, the fever being often just as intense, and the general symptoms just as severe as in the unmodified disease. The difference, however, becomes at once obvious with the appearance of the rash. The pocks are always much fewer than even in mild small-pox, sometimes even not more than twenty. They never attain above half the size of the ordinary small-pox pustules; they run their course and dry off in half the time, and consequently the dangerous fever which accompanies their development in the natural disease is almost or altogether absent in the vast majority of instances.

If vaccination did no more than this it would be hard to overestimate its value, or to praise as it deserves the merit of its discoverer.

=Chicken-Pox= is an ailment of such slight importance that it would scarcely call for notice if it were not that the resemblance of the eruption to that of small-pox sometimes leads to its being mistaken for that disease.

It is highly contagious, and for this reason perhaps it is usually met with in infancy and early childhood. Sometimes, though by no means constantly, the eruption is preceded for twenty-four or thirty-six hours by slight feverishness; but oftener the appearance of the rash is the first indication of anything being the matter. It shows itself in the form of small pimples, which in a few hours change into small circular pocks containing a little slightly turbid fluid. They appear on the forehead, face, and body, but very rarely on the limbs; they enlarge for some two or at most three days, then shrivel and dry up; and at the end of a week the crusts or scabs fall off, scarcely ever causing any permanent pitting of the skin. They are usually not above twenty or thirty in number, though every now and then they are much more numerous without any obvious reason. Their distinction from the small-pox eruption consists not only in the smaller size of the pocks, and in the entirely different course which they run, but also in the fact that two or three successive crops of the eruption appear in the course of five or six days, so that new ones, those at maturity, and those on which the crusts have already formed, or from which they have already fallen, may be seen on the child at the same time. This is sufficient of itself to establish the difference between the two diseases, and also to distinguish between chicken-pox and the milder variety of small-pox which is sometimes observed in children who have been already vaccinated.

=Measles= is a disease with which almost everyone is familiar, and one which with proper care is not generally attended with danger. Its great risks are twofold; first, that of its being complicated with bronchitis, or inflammation of the lungs during its progress, and next of its being followed by an imperfect recovery, and by the awakening into activity any tendency to scrofulous or consumptive disease. On these two accounts the disease is not to be made light of, and special watchfulness is to be exercised during the whole time of convalescence. It is also unwise when one child in a family is attacked by measles to expose the others, as is often done, to its contagion, in order, as people say, 'to get it over;' for its mildness in one case furnishes no guarantee of its mildness in another, and the danger of the disease is almost in exact proportion to the tender age of those who are attacked by it.

The early symptoms of measles are those of a bad feverish cold; the eyes grow red, weak, and watery, and are unable to bear the light, the child sneezes very frequently, sometimes almost every five minutes, and is troubled by a constant short dry cough. About the fourth day, a rash makes its appearance on the face, forehead, and behind the ears, and in the course of the next forty-eight hours travels downwards over the body and limbs, and then in another forty-eight hours it fades in the same way, being at its height on the body when it has already begun to disappear from the face. It first shows itself in the form of small red circular spots, not unlike fleabites, but very slightly raised above the somewhat reddened skin, and looking for a few hours not unlike the very early stages of small-pox, before the eruption has lost the character of minute pimples. On the face the spots sometimes run together, and then form irregular blotches about a third of an inch long by half that breadth; while elsewhere they present an irregular crescentic arrangement. As the rash fades it puts on a dirty yellowish red appearance; the surface of the skin often becomes slightly scurfy, and it continues somewhat stained of a reddish hue for some days after the eruption has disappeared.

The only other point on which it is necessary to dwell is this, that the symptoms do not, as in small-pox, become less severe immediately on the appearance of the eruption, but continue just as troublesome as before for twenty-four hours or more, the voice being hoarse, the cough even more incessant, and the throat often slightly sore and red. Soon, however, improvement becomes apparent, the fever lessens, the cough grows looser; and in less than a fortnight the patient is usually convalescent.

The above is pretty nearly the ordinary course of measles, for we do not meet with that extreme variation in its severity which is observed in scarlatina, where one child will seem scarcely to ail at all, while its brother or sister may be in a state of extreme peril. It is not wise, however, to trust a case even of apparently mild measles to domestic management, for while the cough is troublesome in almost every case, the ear of the experienced doctor is needed to ascertain whether it is merely the cough of irritation which attends the measles, or the graver cough due to bronchitis.

One other caution will not be out of place. The danger of exposure to cold is very real, but that does not necessitate the loading the child with excessive covering, or the abstaining from washing its hands and face. The child should be kept moderately cool; and sponging its hands and face frequently with tepid water soothes it and relieves the painful irritation and itching.

=German Measles.=--There is a disorder which seems to hold a middle place between measles and scarlatina, akin to both, identical with neither, and furnishing no sort of protection from their occurrence.

It is known in this country by the name of German measles, or sometimes by its German name of R 鰐 heln; the first clear description of its character having been given by German writers.

It is unfortunate that a very slight resemblance of some of its symptoms to those of scarlet fever has led to its being sometimes mistaken for it, and as the ailment is almost always very trivial, doctors anxious to avoid alarming their patients' friends, too often allow the error to go unrectified, and the disease to pass as one of mild scarlet fever.

The resemblance of German measles to scarlet fever is, however, extremely slight, and is almost entirely limited to the existence of a slight sore-throat, unaccompanied with glandular swelling. The rash in no respect resembles the uniform redness of the scarlatinal eruption, and there is no peeling of the skin, nor even any roughness of the surface left behind.

Slight feverishness sometimes precedes the appearance of the rash for twenty-four hours; but the cough, and sneezing, and running at the eyes and nose, which usher in measles are entirely absent. The rash usually appears in the course of twenty-four hours, is never postponed beyond the second day; it begins, like that of measles, on the face, and, like it, travels downwards, but always disappears on the third day, while that of measles is not entirely gone before the eighth or ninth. The rash itself also has a different character. It consists of small, slightly elevated, round red spots which now and then coalesce into small patches, but never have the somewhat crescentic arrangement observed in the rash of measles. The colour of the spots is somewhat darker than that of the eruption of measles, while the skin between them remains pale, and does not assume the flush of measles. As it disappears it simply fades, and does not at all change its tint as that of measles does, and it leaves the skin unroughened.

Now and then German measles are severe, and are attended with a good deal of fever for a day or two, and even with symptoms of bronchitis. These cases are, however, very unusual, are seen only at times when the disease prevails epidemically; and even then the symptoms of the affection are sufficiently marked to preserve from error all but those who wish to be deceived, and to flatter themselves that their child is henceforth protected from scarlatina.

=Scarlatina=, or =Scarlet Fever=, for the two names mean the same thing, the former being only the Latin term, and not implying any greater mildness of the disease, is one of the most formidable ailments of childhood, and especially of early childhood, since the highest mortality from it takes place during the third year of life.

It is more dreaded in a household, and justly so, than any other disease of childhood, though, indeed, it is not limited in its occurrence to early life, and instances are familiar to us all in which the mother, devoting herself to the care of her little ones, has herself fallen a victim to the poison.

I do not think it so directly contagious, from person to person, as small-pox, chicken-pox, or measles, but its infection appears to be specially abiding in its character, and to cling longer to the clothes, the bedding, and even the room of a scarlet fever patient, than that of the other eruptive fevers, except perhaps small-pox.

It is an object of special dread also for two other reasons. One of these reasons is the extreme and causeless variations in its severity; so that I have known more than one or two children in the same family to have it so slightly as scarcely to be ill, two to have their lives placed in jeopardy, and two to die. The other reason for special dread is that the mildness of the disease at its outset affords but a slight guarantee against the occurrence of serious complications in its course, and still slighter against secondary diseases which may follow in its train, and either destroy life directly, or leave behind some irremediable mischief.

Scarlatina has been divided by medical men into three classes, according to its different degrees of severity; the mild--that accompanied with bad sore-throat--and the malignant variety.

We have specially to do with the first of the three; for it is in it only that there is danger of the disease being overlooked, or mistaken.

The symptoms of scarlatina usually appear within three days after exposure to its contagion, and there is very good authority for believing that the interval never exceeds six days. I should not, however, feel quite secure until after the lapse of ten days, and during this time the child ought to be isolated from his brothers and sisters. In the mildest form of the disease the appearance of the rash upon the surface, usually with, but sometimes even without slight sore-throat and feverishness, may be the first indication of an affection which is sometimes so deadly. In the majority of cases, however, it is ushered in by vomiting once or oftener, accompanied by headache, heaviness, of head, great heat of skin, and some measure of sore-throat. The brain is easily disturbed in children, as has already been said, and delirium at night during the first twenty-four hours of an attack of scarlet fever need not excite anxiety, for it then often passes away, and the disease runs a perfectly favourable course. The continuance of delirium later is an attendant only on the graver forms of scarlet fever.

The rash often makes its appearance within twenty-four hours after the commencement of the illness, at latest in the course of the second day. It usually shows itself first on the neck, breast, and face, whence it extends in twenty-four hours to the body and limbs, and is then not seldom specially vivid on the inside of the thighs. Its colour is a very bright red, due in part to a general flush of the skin, in part to the presence of innumerable red dots or spots, which do not communicate any sense of roughness to the hand, though now and then extremely minute red pimples are interspersed. For three days the rash usually continues to become of a deeper colour, and more generally diffused over the whole surface; it then slowly declines, but does not wholly disappear until the seventh or eighth day of the disease. As the rash subsides the skin is left rough, and by degrees scales off, often in large flakes from the hands and feet, but elsewhere in a sort of branny scales. Sometimes this process is over in five or six days, while in other cases the skin peels and is reproduced several times in succession, so that it is protracted for three or four weeks or even longer. The degree of this peeling also varies as well as its duration. It is usually most considerable where the rash has been most abundant, while where the rash has been scanty, it is sometimes scarcely apparent except at the tips of the fingers and toes and just around the insertion of the nails.

Besides the rash there are commonly other symptoms not less characteristic of scarlatina, and among them the sore-throat is one of the most invariable.

Even in mild cases, it is very rarely absent, and if not present at the beginning, it comes on on the second or third day. The palate and tonsils, in these circumstances are red, and the latter are usually more or less swollen, while swallowing is attended with pain, or at any rate with discomfort. The redness of the palate, which extends also to the back of the throat, is a finely spotted redness closely resembling the rash on the surface. The tongue is coated with a thick white or yellowish coating, through which project numerous bright red points, papill?as they are called, and this appearance of the tongue is as distinctive of scarlatina as the rash itself. Later, as the rash begins to fade, the coating separates from the tongue, which is left of a bright red colour, looking raw and shining, with the little raised red points projecting beyond its surface, and constituting what has been called in medical language, the strawberry tongue.

When all these symptoms are present, no one can doubt but that the case is one of scarlatina. But the decision is far less easy in mild cases, for in them the rash is sometimes extremely evanescent, the general disturbance of health very slight, and the fever and accompanying rise of temperature small. The risk in such circumstances of the disease being altogether overlooked is even greater than that of its being confounded with some other eruptive fever. The rash of measles cannot be confounded with that of scarlatina, and the distinctly spotty character of the rash of German measles ought, apart even from other differences, to render mistake impossible.

Perhaps the best rule that can be laid down is that every diffused red rash, not obviously formed by distinct spots, even though it be not uniform but appears in patches on the neck, breast, back, or inside of the thighs, and persists for more than twelve hours, is scarlatinal. Further, that in any instance in which even very slight feverishness, or very slight sore-throat, have preceded or accompanied the rash, the nature of the ailment is stamped beyond the possibility of doubt. Mistakes are made from want of careful observation, much more than from any insuperable difficulty in distinguishing one disease from the other. When the least hesitation is felt as to the nature of any rash which may appear on a child, with, or without previous illness, the question should be at once referred to a medical man. People are too apt in these circumstances to wait for a few days, and then to appeal to the doctor when all traces of rash have disappeared, and when the grounds no longer exist on which he could base a positive opinion.

I need not describe the symptoms of severe and dangerous scarlatina, for long before symptoms become really formidable, the patients will have been placed under medical care. It may suffice to say that the danger is almost always in proportion to the severity of the throat-affection and swelling of the glands, and not at all in proportion to the abundance of the rash. Though severe cases usually set in with severe symptoms, yet this is not invariably the case, and medical watching is all the more necessary from the very commencement, since until the end of the first week it is impossible to calculate on the subsequent course of the disease. In malignant scarlatina happily of infrequent occurrence, the child is struck down, as though its blood were poisoned, from the very first; and death takes place often within forty-eight hours, the rash appearing just sufficiently to stamp the nature of the pestilence which has proved so deadly.

It may form a useful conclusion to all that has been said in this little book about the diseases of children, if I endeavour to point out in what consist the duties of parents in cases of scarlatina, or of any disease which resembles it.

1. To watch carefully the commencement of every slight feverish attack in which a diffused red rash appears, even though this should be only in patches, and to bear in mind the possibility of its being due to scarlatina.

2. To remove the child immediately from the others, so long as there is any doubt concerning the nature of the case, and to remove with him his bed, bedding, and all clothes worn by him at the time when the illness began, or the rash appeared.

3. To place the child if possible in a room at the top of the house, so that the other children may not pass by his door.

4. Inasmuch as scarlatina often proves fatal to grown persons who have not already had the disease, to obtain at once the attendance of a skilled nurse, in order to avoid the risk of the disease spreading through the household.

The wife belongs to her husband, the husband to his wife; their mutual duties are paramount over even those of the parent; and neither has the right to jeopardise that life which belongs to the other. To say, 'I shall not catch the disease, because I have no fear,' is as idle as it would be for the soldier to say, 'Because I am brave, therefore I am invulnerable.'

I have been accustomed to insist on the absence from the room of father or mother, supposing either of them not to have had scarlatina, so long as I could give the assurance that every thing was going on well; but on the slightest anxiety I have referred to both parents for their mutual decision as to the course which they would choose to adopt.

From a refusal to be guided by this counsel, it has more than once happened to me, to see the child recover from mild scarlatina without a bad symptom, and the mother who had insisted on nursing the little one die of the disease to which she had needlessly exposed herself.

5. So soon as the disease has declared itself as scarlatina, to take up the carpets and remove the curtains from the sick child's room, to empty the drawers of any clothes which may be in them, and to hang up outside the door a sheet moistened with a solution of carbolic acid.

6. To arrange for all food and necessaries to be placed in an adjoining room, or at the head of the stairs, so that there may be no direct communication between the attendants on the sick and the other inmates of the house.

7. To insist on the attendants not wearing either silk or stuff dresses, but dresses of some washable material; and on their changing their garments as well as scrupulously washing themselves before mixing with other inmates of the house, and especially with the children.

8. While in all respects obeying the directions of the doctor, to grease the child all over twice in twenty-four hours with suet or lard, to which a small quantity of carbolic acid has been added. This proceeding both lessens the amount of peeling of the skin in a later stage of the disease; lessens the contagiousness of the scales which are detached; and, by promoting the healthy action of the skin, diminishes the risk of subsequent disorder of the kidneys and consequent dropsy.

9. Even when the case has been of the slightest possible kind, to keep the child always in bed for one-and-twenty days. This was a standing rule at the

Children's Hospital, and I am certain that its non-observance will be followed three times out of four by dropsy and kidney-disease.

10. When the disease is over, to destroy, if the parents' means at all permit it, the clothes and bedding of the child. When this is not practicable, to have everything exposed to the heat of superheated steam in a Washington Lyons or other similar disinfector, and to have all linen boiled as well as washed. Lastly, to have the ceiling whitewashed, the paint cleaned, the paper stripped, and the room repapered, as well as the floor washed and rewashed with strong carbolic soap.

These precautions are troublesome and costly, but disease is costlier still; and who shall estimate the cost of death!

APPENDIX

ON THE MENTAL AND MORAL FACULTIES IN CHILDHOOD, AND ON THE DISORDERS TO WHICH THEY ARE LIABLE.

Any remarks on the ailments of children would be incomplete if no notice were taken of the mental and moral peculiarities of early life.

For want of giving heed to them, not only are grave mistakes made in the education of children, but in the management of their ailments, both by doctors and by parents: much needless trouble is given to the doctors, much needless distress to the child, much needless anxiety to the parents.

The common mistake committed by those parents who do not make their child an idol to fall down and worship, and thus turn him, to his own misery and theirs, into the most arbitrary of domestic tyrants, is to treat him as though he were in mind, as well as in body, a miniature man; feebler in intellect as he is inferior in strength, but differing in degree only, not in kind.

Now the child differs essentially from the adult in the three respects; that

1. He lives in the present, not in the future.

2. His perceptions are more vivid, and his sensibilities more acute; while the

world, on which he has just entered, surrounds him with daily novelties.

3. He has less self-consciousness, less self-dependence, lives as a part of the world by which he is surrounded--a real practical pantheist.

The child lives in the present, not in the future, nor much even in the past, till the world has been some time with him, and he by degrees shares the common heritage of retrospect and anticipation. This is the great secret of the quiet happiness which strikes almost all visitors to a children's hospital.

No one can have watched the sick bed of the child without remarking the almost unvarying patience with which its illness is borne, and the extremity of peril from which apparently, in consequence of that patience, a complete recovery takes place. Much, indeed, is no doubt due to the activity of the reparative powers in early life, but much also to the unruffled quiet of the mind. No sorrow for the past, no gloomy foreboding of the future, no remorse, disappointment, nor anxiety depresses the spirits and enfeebles the vital powers. The prospect of death, even when its approach is realised--and this is not so rare as some may imagine--brings in general but small alarm. This may be from the vagueness of the child's ideas; it may be, as the poet says, that in his short life's journey, 'the heaven that lies about us in our infancy' has been so much with him, that he recognises more clearly than we can do

'The glories he hath known, And that imperial palace whence he came.'

I dwell on this truth, because it is of great practical moment that we should bear in mind to how very large an extent the child lives only in the present; because it follows from it that to keep the sick child happy; to remove from it all avoidable causes of alarm, of suffering, of discomfort; to avoid, as far as may be, any direct struggle with its waywardness; and even if death seems likely to occur, to look at it from a child's point of view--not from that which our larger understanding of good and evil suggests to our minds--are duties of the gravest kind which weigh on the parent and the nurse, no less than on the physician.

But not only does the child live in the present far more than it is possible for the adult, but there are, besides, other important mental differences between the two. Not only is the mind of the child feebler in all respects than that of the adult, but, in proportion to the feebleness of his reasoning power, there is an exaggerated activity of his perceptive faculties, a vividness of his imagination. The child lives at first in the external world, as if it were a part of himself, or he a part of it, and the gladheartedness which it rejoices us to see is as much a result of the vividness with which he realises the things around him, as of that absence of care to which it is often attributed. This peculiarity shows itself in the dreams of childhood, which exceed in the distinctness of their images those which come in later life. It shows itself, too, in the frequency with which, even when awake, the active organs perceive unreal sounds, or in the dark, at night, conjure up ocular spectra; and then not merely colours, but distinct shapes, which pass in long procession before the eyes. This power fades away with advancing life; except under some conditions of disease, the occasional appearance of luminous objects in the dark is the only relic with most of us of the gift of seeing visions with which, at least in some degree, we were endowed in our early years. The child who dreads to be alone, and asserts that he hears sounds, or perceives objects, is not expressing merely a vague apprehension of some unknown danger, but often asserts a literal truth. The sounds have been heard; in the stillness of its nursery the little one has listened to what seemed a voice calling it; or, in the dark, phantasms have risen before its eyes, and the agony of terror with which it calls for a light, or begs for its mother's presence, betrays an impression far too real to be explained away, or to be met by hard words or by unkind treatment.

Impressions such as these are not uncommon in childhood, even during health. Disorder, direct or indirect, of the functions of the brain, more commonly the latter, greatly exaggerates them, and I have known them to outlast for many weeks all other signs of failing health after convalescence from fevers. The unreal sights are far more common than the sounds. The sounds are usually of the simplest kind--as the tinkling of a bell, of which we all remember the exquisite use made by Hans Andersen in one of his nursery tales; or the child's own name, at intervals repeated, just as the little watchful boy heard it in far off Judea, when it was the prelude to a wondrous communication from the unseen world. It came to him as he woke from sleep, before the morning dawned, while the lamp, lighted overnight, was burning still; and still it is so far the same that these occurrences which suggest to us problems that we cannot attempt to solve, mostly take place at times of transition from the sleeping to the waking state.

The ocular spectra are usually far more vivid and detailed. Those which occur in the waking state are by no means always painful, though their strangeness not infrequently alarms the child, and his horror at the dark arises, not from his seeing nothing, but from his seeing too much.

Some imaginative children amuse themselves with these phantasms, and then, if encouraged to relate them, will constantly transgress the boundary line between truth and falsehood, and weave their little romance. When they happen on waking they are usually preceded by frightful dreams, but the image which the child sees then is not the mere recollection of the dream, but a new, distinct, though painful impression; generally of some animal to which the child points, as now here, now there. These night terrors from the very circumstantial character of the impressions which attend them, often, as I have already said, occasion needless anxiety as to the importance of the cause on which they depend.

Sleep-walking in its smaller degrees of getting out of bed at night, is by no means unusual in childhood; but the greater degrees of somnambulism are certainly rare; and I have always found them dependent on undue mental work; not always, indeed, on the tasks being excessive, but sometimes on the over-anxiety of the child to make progress. I have not yet known a poor person's child a somnambulist.

But not only are the perceptions more acute in childhood than in adult life, the sensibilities are more intense. The child's emotions, indeed, are often transitory--generally very transitory; but while they last they produce results far greater than in the grown person. In the case of the latter, recollection of the past, anticipation of the future, or even the duties of the present, control the overwhelming sorrow, or call forth the energies needed to bear it. The child lives in the present, and this present is but the reflection of the world around, its impressions uncontrolled by experience, ungoverned by reason.

The broken-heartedness of a child on leaving home is not the expression only of intense affection for its friends or relations, it is the shock of separation from the familiar objects which have surrounded it; and I have not infrequently seen children inconsolable when removed from homes that were most wretched, or from relations who were most unkind. Every now and then, indeed, I have been compelled to send children home from the hospital because no love nor care could reconcile them to the change from home; and they have refused to eat, and spent their nights in weeping. The feeling is an unreasoning one, like the home-sickness of the mountaineer.

But, moreover, sudden shocks may sometimes overthrow the whole moral equilibrium, and disarrange the balance of the nervous system so seriously as to cause the death of a child previously free from any important ailment. Thus, I remember a little boy five years of age who died sixteen days after his father's funeral. The strange sad scene overcame him, though there had been no special tie between him and his father. He shivered violently, became very sick, complained by signs of pain in the head, for he had lost his speech, which he regained by slow degrees in the course of four or five days. Improvement in other respects did not take place, he lay in a drowsy state save when he called for his mother, and at length the drowsiness deepened into stupor, and so he died. I suppose his mother was right; she said his heart was broken.

It behoves us to bear in mind that the heart may break, or the reason fail, under causes that seem to us quite insufficient; that the griefs of childhood may be, in proportion to the child's powers of bearing them, as overwhelming as those which break the strong man down. Every now and then we are shocked by the tale that some young child has committed suicide, and for reasons which to our judgment seem most trivial--from fear of punishment, or even from mere dread of reproof. These facts deserve special attention, they show how much more the susceptibility and sensitiveness of children need to be taken into consideration than is commonly done.

This keenness of the emotions in children displays itself in other ways, and has constantly to be borne in mind in our management of them. The child loves intensely, or dislikes strongly; craves most earnestly for sympathy, clings most tenaciously to the stronger, better, higher around it, or to what it fancies so; or shrinks, in often causeless but unconquerable dread, from things or persons that have made on it an unpleasant impression. Reason as yet does not govern its caprices, nor the more intelligent selfishness of later years hinder their manifestation. The waywardness of the most wilful child is determined by some cause near at hand; and those who love children, and can read their thoughts, will not in general be long in discovering their motives and seeing through their conduct.

One word more must be said with reference to that intense craving for sympathy so characteristic of the child. It is this which often underlies the disposition to exaggerate its ailments, or even to feign such as do not exist, and in such attempts at deception it often perseveres with almost incredible resolution. Over and over again I have met with instances where the motives to such deception were neither the increase of comfort nor the gratification of mere indolence; but the monopolising the love and sympathy which during some bygone illness had been extended to it, and which it could not bear to share again with its brothers and sisters. This feeling, too, sometimes becomes quite uncontrollable, and the child then needs as much care and as judicious management, both bodily and mental, to bring it back to health, as would be called for in the case of some adult hypochondriac or monomaniac.

A caution may not be out of place as to the importance of not ministering to this tendency to exaggerated self-consciousness by talking of children's ailments in their hearing, or by seeming to notice the complaints they make as though they were something out of the common way.

It will be observed that throughout I have dwelt more on disorders of the moral faculties than of the intellectual powers in childhood, and I have done so because I believe them to be the more common and the more important. In the feeble-minded the moral sense almost invariably participates in the weakness of the intellect; but it is by no means unusual for the former to be grievously perverted, while the intelligence is in no respect deficient. The moral element in the child seems to me to assert its superiority in this, that it is the most keenly sensitive, the soonest disordered--

'Like sweet bells jangled, out of tune, and harsh,'

and the discord is first perceived in the finest notes.

To a very great extent, a mixture of vanity and of a morbid craving for sympathy lie at the root of many of those perversions of character which excite a parent's anxiety. One of these consists in an over-scrupulousness with reference to the right or wrong of actions in themselves quite indifferent;

in doubts as to whether the morning or evening prayer has been properly said, whether something was or was not absolutely true, whether this or that peccadillo was a grievous offence against God, and so on; and all these little cases of conscience are brought by the child several times a day to his mother or to his nurse for solution. If listened to readily the child's truthfulness becomes inevitably destroyed, and he grows up with a morbid frame of mind, which after-life will aggravate almost infinitely.

One knows indeed the history of child saints; but it must be remembered that one great characteristic of pre-eminent sanctity at all ages of life is reticence, while these little people are perpetually seeking to interest others in themselves, their doubts, and feelings. If wisely dealt with, not by direct ridicule, but by a wholesome neglect of the child's revelations, treating them as of no special interest or importance, and discouraging that minute introspection which, of doubtful good at any age, is absolutely destructive of the simplicity of childhood, this unnatural condition will soon pass away. It will help this object very much, if the child is sent on a visit to judicious friends, and change of scene, of pursuits, of playmates, and amusements will be of all the more service since these morbid states of mind seldom come on in children whose bodily health is robust.

Another mode in which the same perverted feelings display themselves is in the disposition occasionally noticed to exaggerate some real ailment, or to complain of some ailment which is altogether imaginary. So far is this from being rare that my experience coincides entirely with that of the French physician M. Roger, who has had larger opportunities than anyone else in France for observing the diseases of children, and who says, 'It must be borne in mind that simulated ailments are much more common in the children's hospital than in a hospital for adults.'

It is difficult to assign any sufficient reason for this conduct. Mere indolence seems sometimes to be the chief reason for it, oftener vanity; the sense of importance in finding everything in the household arranged with exclusive reference to itself appears to be the motive for it; and this may sometimes be observed to be very powerful even at an exceedingly early age. In many instances a morbid craving for sympathy is mingled with the love of importance, and both these sentiments are not infrequently exaggerated by the conduct of a foolishly fond mother. Real illness, however, in almost all these cases exists at the commencement, though the child persists in complaining of its old symptoms long after their cause has disappeared.

The great difficulty which the doctor meets with in the management of these cases arises from the incredulity with which his opinion is received. Candour is looked upon as so eminently characteristic of childhood, that deceit seems impossible; the case is thought by the parents to be an obscure one which the doctor does not understand; and therefore it is said, he, with want of straightforwardness and of kindness, throws doubts on the existence of disease, and on the truthfulness of a most loving, most suffering child. The vagaries of a hysterical girl, the fits, the palsy, the half-unconsciousness have all been assumed within my own observation by children from ten to fifteen years old, and I have more than once had to give place to the ignorant and impudent pretender who traded successfully on the feelings of the parents. Sometimes, one knows not why, except that the child has got tired of the part he was playing, the symptoms that had caused so much anxiety suddenly disappear, but even then the habit of mind left behind is anything but healthy. Indeed in all cases of this kind it is much less the state of the body than that of the mind which excites my apprehension. The constant watching its own sensations, the habit of constantly gratifying every wayward wish and temper under the plea of illness, and the constant indulgence which it too often meets with in this from the over-kindness of its parents, exert a most injurious influence on its character, and it grows up a juvenile hypochondriac.

A doctor is very unlikely to throw doubt recklessly on the reality of a child's illness. His hesitation should certainly not be attributed to unworthy motives; the parents should co-operate with him heartily in any course of observation which he desires to follow, and if necessary another medical man of experience should be associated with the first, and allowed to visit the child two or three times. One does not associate the idea of moral delinquency with hysteria; the child who shams belongs to the same class with the hysterical patient. It is only the strangeness of the occurrence in the eyes of non-medical people, that makes them fancy it something worse.

If now the suspicion is justified that the child is either greatly exaggerating or altogether feigning illness, it does not by any means always follow that he should at once be charged with it, since it is often of much importance that his self-respect should not be destroyed. It must be remembered that there is in all these cases a measure of real ailment underlying all the half-unconscious exaggeration, and that if spoiling and over-indulgence do much to foster it, sternness and punishment interfere with recovery. To turn the thoughts away from self, to occupy the mind with new scenes, new amusements, new pursuits, to call forth by degrees self-control, and to let the child perceive rather by your manner than by what is actually said that the parents have not been duped by all his past vagaries; such are the simple means by which the little one will be brought round again to health of mind and health of body. Unhappily, in the minds of too many people the idea of the doctor is associated with the administration of drugs and with nothing else; the treatment of disease is of much wider scope; and many of our best remedies are those which do not admit of being weighed or measured, and whose names are not inscribed on the drawers or bottles in Apothecaries' Hall.

Another phase of mental disorder in childhood sometimes presents itself as the result of overtasking the intellectual powers. This over-work too is by no means due in all cases to the parents' unwisely urging the child forward, but it is often quite voluntary on his part. The precaution too of limiting the hours of work is often inadequate from the want of some provision for turning the thoughts and energies during play hours into some perfectly different channel.

In many of these cases Nature happily takes matters into her own management. For a year or two, or more, the mind has grown apparently at the expense of the body; the parents take a fearful joy in their darling's acquirements; and if it should live, think they, of what remarkable talents will it not be the possessor! By degrees, the extreme quickness of intellect becomes less remarkable; but the body begins to increase in robustness; and a year will sometimes suffice to transmute the little fairy, so quick, so clever, but so fragile, into a very commonplace, merry, rosy, romping child. I may add that it is well to bear in mind the converse of this; to remember that body and mind rarely grow in equal proportion at one time; that the incorrigible little dunce, though not likely to prove a genius as he grows older, will yet very probably be found at twelve or fourteen to know as much as his playmates. A dull mind, and a sickly or ill-developed frame may make us anxious: but if the physical development is good, the mind will not be likely to remain long below the average standard.

But sometimes, the over-tasked mind leads to mischief which Nature cannot rectify; an attack of water on the brain destroys the child, or if not it sinks under almost any accidental disease. In other instances neither of these results takes place, but the whole nervous system seems profoundly shaken, and the moral character of the child seriously, and even permanently injured. I remember a quick and clever little girl aged five and a half years who was urged on by her governess to work which she delighted in, till at length the signs of over-taxed brain showed themselves in frequent extreme irritability, and occasional attacks of causeless fury amounting almost to madness. It was fully a year during which almost all mental work was suspended, while the child was sent to have complete change under most judicious management in the country, before her mind quite recovered its balance and she became able to resume her studies in a very moderate degree.

Cases such as this are instances of the slightest degree of a condition which if not remedied may pass into confirmed insanity. I believe the gradations to be almost imperceptible by which the one state passes into the other; and I have known instances in which the ungovernable temper and occasional fury of the child have passed in youth into abiding insanity which rendered the patient the inmate, and I fear the permanent inmate, of a lunatic asylum.

In whatever circumstances insanity comes on in childhood, and it does sometimes, though very seldom, come on independently of any obvious exciting cause, it always assumes the character of what has been termed moral insanity, or of that condition in which the moral system rather than the mental power is chiefly disordered.

Idiocy is unquestionably of much more frequent occurrence in childhood, than any of those forms of mental or moral disorder of which I have been speaking hitherto. The term idiocy, however, is a very wide one, including conditions differing remarkably from each other both in kind and degree, while not seldom it is misapplied to cases in which there is mere backwardness of intellectual power.

=Backward Children.=-constitute a class by no means seldom met with. They generally attain their bodily development slowly, and the development of their mind is equally tardy. They cut their teeth late, walk late, talk late, are slow in learning to wash and dress themselves, are generally dull in their perceptions, and do not lay aside the habits of infancy till far advanced in childhood. When the time comes for positive instruction, their slowness almost wears out everyone's patience; and among the poor indeed the attempt at teaching such children is at length given up in despair, and growing up in absolute ignorance, it is no wonder that they should be regarded as idiots. Still, dull as such children are, there is between them and the idiot an essential difference. The backward child, unlike the idiot, does not remain stationary; his development goes on, but more slowly than that of other children, he is behind them in the whole course of their progress, and his delay increasing every day, places at length an enormous distance between him and them--a distance which in fact becomes insurmountable.

In some of its minor degrees even, this backwardness not infrequently excites the solicitude of parents. It is sometimes observed in children who had been ill-nourished in infancy or who had been weakened by some serious or protracted illness, even though unattended by any special affection of the brain; but it is also met with independent of any special cause. The distinction, however, between such a case and one of idiocy is this, that though at four years old the child may not seem to be intellectually superior to most children at two, yet in manners, habits, and intelligence it does agree with what might be expected from the child at two; less bright perhaps, less joyous, but still presenting nothing which if it were but younger would awaken apprehension.

It is well in all cases of unusual backwardness to ascertain the condition of the sense of hearing, and of the power of speech, for I have known the existence of deafness long overlooked, and the child's dulness and inability to speak referred to intellectual deficiency; and have also observed mere difficulty of articulation, dependent partly on malformation of the mouth, lead to a similar misapprehension. In both instances I have seen this inability to keep up ready intercourse with other children cast a shadow over the mind, and the little ones in consequence be dull, suspicious, unchild-like. I have already referred to a similar result as sometimes following serious illnesses. The child will for months cease to walk, or forget to talk, if these had been but comparatively recent acquirements; or will continue dull and unequal to any mental effort for weeks or months together, and then the mind will begin to develop itself once more, though slowly, possibly so slowly as never altogether to make up for lost ground.

=Idiocy.=--In idiocy, however, there is much more than the mere arrest of the intellect at any period. The idiot of eight years old does not correspond in his mental development to the child at six, or four, or two; his mind is not only dwarfed but deformed; while feebleness of will is often as remarkable as mere deficiency of power of apprehension. Even in earliest infancy there is usually a something in the child idiotic from birth which marks him as different from babies of his own age. He is unable to support his head, which rolls about from side to side, almost without an effort on his part to prevent it. Next it is perceived that the child, though he can see, does not notice; that his eye does not meet his mother's with the fond look of recognition, accompanied with the dimpling smile, with which the infant, even of three months old, greets his mother. Then it is found to have no notion of grasping anything, though that is usually almost the first accomplishment of babyhood; if tossed in its nurse's arms there seems to be no spring in its limbs; and though a strange vacant smile sometimes passes over its face, yet the merry ringing laugh of infancy or joyous chuckle of irrepressible glee is not heard. As time passes on, the child shows no pleasure at being put down 'to feel its feet,' as nurses term it; if laid on the floor it probably cries, but does not attempt to turn round, nor try to crawl about as other babies do. It does not learn to stand or walk till late, and then stands awkwardly, walks with difficulty, crossing its legs immediately on assuming the erect posture, an infirmity which it often takes years to overcome. Just, too, as the idiot is slow to notice, slow in learning to grasp anything, or to stand or walk, so he is late in learning to talk, he often acquires but few words, for his ideas are few. He learns even these few with difficulty, and employs the same to express many different things; he generally articulates them indistinctly, often indeed so imperfectly as to be almost unintelligible.

In other instances the evidences of idiocy are not present at birth, or at any rate are not then noticed, but succeed to some attack of convulsions or to some illness attended with serious affection of the brain. Sometimes too there is no point in the child's history which can be laid hold on as marking the commencement of the weakening of his intellect, but as the body grows the mind remains stationary, or its powers retrocede, until by degrees the painful conviction that the child has become idiotic forces itself upon the unwilling parents. Here we have sometimes the sad spectacle of the body perfectly developed, hale and strong, but the mind obscured; the child in constant unrest, perpetually chattering, laughing without cause, destroying its clothes, or the furniture of its room, for no purpose; or sitting silent, with a weird smile upon its face, looking at its spread-out fingers, or stroking a piece of cloth for a quarter of an hour together as though the sensation yielded it a kind of pleasure. It would be almost endless to describe the various degrees of mental weakness; from the slight silliness down to the condition in which the child is, and remains all life long, below the level of the brute.

Parents as a rule are anxious to persuade themselves, and to persuade the doctor that their idiot child was once as bright and intelligent as others; and that the mind was darkened by some grave illness. We have, however, the highest authority, that of Dr. Down, for saying that as a rule which has but few exceptions idiocy from birth is more amenable to training than that which comes on afterwards, that in fact it is more hopeful to have to do with an ill-developed than with a damaged brain.

The one great question which still remains is what can the parents do for best and wisest whom the affliction has befallen of having an idiot child.

First. To moderate their expectations as to the results of any, even the best devised and most successful treatment. The child who has been born of weak intellect, or who has become so as the result of illness, will always remain at a lower level than others, and this, even though some one faculty, as the musical faculty, or the power of calculation, should be above the average.

Secondly. From the child's earliest infancy to occupy themselves in perfecting as far as possible the physical powers and aptitudes, and the habits of cleanliness and order. Development of mind waits on development of body: to stand, to sit, to walk, to grasp an object put into the hand, are essential to bringing the idiot child into relation with the world around it; are its elementary education, to be given patiently, cheerfully, lovingly, even for years together. To attend to its natural wants, and by fixed routine to accustom it at stated hours to empty its bowels and its bladder is a lesson hard to teach; and not less difficult is it to make the child learn to masticate its food, to drink without slobbering, and then to use the spoon and fork, and to feed itself; and afterwards to dress itself, to wash itself, to tie its shoestrings; for idiots almost without exception are awkward as well as lazy.

The common class of nurses, even the very kindest, find it so much easier to feed the child, to wash it, and to dress it, than to teach it to do any of these things for itself, that it too often grows up, till too old to remain in the nursery, without having made the slightest advance above the condition of completest babyhood. It is absolutely essential either that the mother should devote herself solely to the care and teaching of the idiot, or that she should engage a nurse who will have no other duty. Such a person must be above the average in education and intelligence, and of course will command more than the ordinary wages. The mother, too, must resign herself to the little one's affection being transferred in a great degree from herself to the person who has constant charge of it--a hard trial this, but one to which, for her child's good, she must bring herself to submit.

Thirdly. So soon as the child has been taught at home to exercise these lower powers, and the question of what is termed its education arises, it is a matter of absolute necessity that he be sent to an institution specially set apart for the feeble-minded. It is absolutely impossible with the most devoted love and the most lavish expenditure of money, to do at home what can be, and is constantly, accomplished even in a pauper idiot asylum. The imitative faculty, which is usually very strongly marked in the idiot, furnishes one great means of his improvement; while besides there are many of the moral powers which cannot be brought out except in the society of other children of his own age and not differing too widely from him in mental power.

I have warned, and I repeat the warning, against exaggerated expectations as to the results of even the wisest treatment. To teach cleanliness, order, and neatness; to impart knowledge enough to enable the idiot to take care of himself; to develop his affections; to enable him to read and write; to practise some easy handicraft; to partake of some simple pleasures, and so at length to return to the shelter of his own home, and to be there, not an object to be hidden away, too painful to look upon, but an object rather of special tenderness, repaying with his guileless love the sad self-sacrifice of his parents for many a year; these are endeavours almost sure of accomplishment in a well-conducted institution, sure never to be realised in a home.

I have often sent afflicted parents, who shrank from parting with their children, to one institution near London; and I doubt not there are others in England, where pains, and care, and skill, and untiring love awake the slumbering intellect, arouse the dormant affections, and work miracles of healing on these helpless little ones.

###

www.ingramcontent.com/pod-product-compliance
Lightning Source LLC
Chambersburg PA
CBHW070855180526
45168CB00005B/1822